PHARMACY EDUCATION
Teaching and Research Guide

PHARMACY EDUCATION

Teaching and Research Guide

Kashappa Goud H. Desai, M. Pharm., Ph. D
Department Pharmaceutical Sciences
College of Pharmacy
University of Michigan
Ann Arbor, Michigan, USA

ANMOL PUBLICATIONS PVT. LTD.
NEW DELHI - 110 002 (INDIA)

ANMOL PUBLICATIONS PVT. LTD.
H.O.: 4374/4B, Ansari Road, Daryaganj,
New Delhi-110002 (India)
Ph.: 23278000, 23261597
B.O.: No. 1015, Ist Main Road, BSK IIIrd Stage
IIIrd Phase, IIIrd Block,
Bangalore - 560 085 (India)
Visit us at: www.anmolpublications.com

Pharmacy Education: Teaching and Research Guide

First Edition, 2009

ISBN 978-81-261-4063-3

PRINTED IN INDIA

Printed at Balaji Offset, Delhi.

Dedicated to
My Father,
Mother and Siblings

CONTENTS

Foreword *xi*

Preface *xiii*

Acknowledgements *xvii*

List of Contributors *xviii*

Section I
TEACHING-LEARNING

1. Teaching Philosophy 3
   Kashappa Goud H. Desai

2. Pharmacy Professionalism 12
   Kashappa Goud H. Desai

3. Teaching-Learning Methods 20
   Kashappa Goud H. Desai

4. Interactive Lecture—A Better Approach and Ways to Perform 22
   Kashappa Goud H. Desai

5. Problem Based Teaching-Learning: Benefits, Process, Responsibilities and Innovations 39
   Shobha Churi

6. Case Based Teaching-Learning 61
   Shobha Churi

7. Electronic (e)-Teaching-Learning Basics and Methods 77
Kashappa Goud H. Desai

8. Information and Communication Technologies in Pharmacy Education: Need, Vision, Goals and Ways to Achieve 81
Kashappa Goud H. Desai

9. Teaching-Learning with Information and Communication Technologies: Integration and Evaluation 96
Kashappa Goud H. Desai

10. Impact of Information and Communication Technologies on Students, Teachers and Educational Institutions 112
Kashappa Goud H. Desai

11. Computer Assisted Teaching-Learning 124
Kashappa Goud H. Desai

12. Web Based Teaching-Learning 139
Kashappa Goud H. Desai

13. Online Teaching-Learning 154
Kashappa Goud H. Desai

14. Mobile Teaching-Learning 168
Kashappa Goud H. Desai

15. Pharmacy Informatics 181
Shobha Churi

16. Traditional and Modern Teaching-Learning Media/Aids 193
Shobha Churi

17. Fundamentals of Student's Performance Evaluation 213
Shobha Churi

Section II
RESEARCH

18. Good Educational Research Process 227
Kashappa Goud H. Desai

19. Basic Research Skills, Ways to Develop and Assessment 237
Kashappa Goud H. Desai

20. Basics of Guiding/Mentoring Students 247
Kashappa Goud H. Desai

21. Art of Writing Good Scientific Manuscript/Paper 254
Kashappa Goud H. Desai

22. Art of Writing a Good Thesis/Dissertation 265
Kashappa Goud H. Desai

23 How to Transform a Thesis to Manuscript(s) 277
Kashappa Goud H. Desai

Index 282

FOREWORD

Education technology has undergone rapid metamorphosis in last one decade. Pharmacy education, as an integral component of health sciences, has witnessed sea change in recent years due to advent of computer applications and e-learning methodology.

The teacher of today has to be a life-long learner and an educator *par excellence.* He has to keep pace with changing trends in his profession. In his book entitled "Pharmacy Education-Teaching and Research Guide", Dr. Kashappa Goud H. Desai, as an experienced educator and researcher in pharmacy, has sincerely attempted to highlight the importance of consolidating teaching-learning process in pharmacy institutions for better dissemination of the knowledge. The emphasis has been laid by him and his colleague Mrs. Shobha Churi on interactive and problem based teaching-learning, pharmacy informatics, online and mobile teaching-learning, good educational research process, art of writing manuscript, thesis and a research paper and several other facets of teaching-learning and evaluation.

Quality teaching in pharmacy is the need of the hour. The key for success of an institution lies in quality of teachers recruited. This book of Dr. Desai shall be certainly an useful guide for all those teachers who wish to excel in the profession of teaching.

I congratulate Dr. Kashappa Goud H. Desai for bringing out a very useful book for strengthening the cause of pharmacy education.

Prof. (Dr.) Chandrakant Kokate, M. Pharm., Ph. D.
Vice-Chancellor
KLE University, Belgaum, Karnataka, India.
Former President, Pharmacy Council of India;
Former Vice-Chancellor, Kakatiya University &
Chairman, All India Board of Pharmacy, A.I.C.T.E.

PREFACE

"Though I never arrived at the perfection I had been so ambitious of obtaining, but fell far short of it, yet I was, by the endeavor, a better and happier man than I otherwise should have been if I had not attempted it."

—Benjamin Franklin

What an inspiring statement! Most of the pharmacy educational institutions in India framed "vision 2020" in 1990s. A question that every educators need to ask now is "have we done enough changes/improvements in the ways we have been teaching to achieve vision 2020"? It's not an easy path for the educational institutions to accomplish a vision 2020. Every educational institution will have to encounter unexpected situations and challenges along the way. Therefore, all the institutions need to "move forward with strong and active faith" in order to successfully forge the path to 2020.

"The only limit to our realization of tomorrow will be our doubts of today. Let us move forward with strong and active faith."

—Franklin Delano Roosevelt

Over the couple of decades, numerous information and communication technologies (ICTs) have been adopted in teaching-learning methodologies across the globe. These technologies not only revolutionized the traditional teaching-learning methods but also provided new modes for teaching-learning the complex subject/topics of pharmacy curriculum. With a constantly evolving education technology, if we envisage the scenario in 2020, the roles and responsibilities of faculty in 2020 will likely be distinctly different than they perform today.

The primary forces that will impact future pharmacy faculty roles and responsibilities are the expectation of efficiency (the need for a more efficient delivery of education is being driven by demand for higher education is already increasing and nontraditional students who are seeking new careers and lifelong learning will continue to increase in numbers), efficacy (the need for more effective/innovative teaching-learning strategies), and excellence (need for 'excellence' at both the higher and professional education levels of accreditation) by our stakeholders. The continuing evolution of educational technology which promotes self-directed learning and assessment is a common thread across all three of these primary forces and its momentum will significantly facilitate success of all three factors.

Educational technology will continue to evolve and become easier to access and use. Educators will have to turn to it as a means for handling larger numbers of students in a more efficient manner. For teaching-learning to be more effective, faculty will continue to find a greater variety of effective teaching-learning and assessment methods. If educators are "evidence-based" in selecting the teaching-learning and assessment strategies for pharmacy students, educators will be using the most efficient and effective instructional methods and therefore be more likely to demonstrate "excellence." With these demands, pharmacy educators will be forced to revise the existing teaching-learning methodologies and also adopt ICTs-based teaching-learning methodologies in their curriculum to prepare future professionals (vision 2020).

Since there has been a growing demand for the paradigm shift in pharmacy academia, I felt that it is necessary to address the traditional teaching-learning methods along with corresponding revolutions. Further, I also felt that there is a need to get an overview on "role of ICTs in pharmacy teaching-learning and functioning of ICTs-based teaching-learning methods". I found that there are no books which include recent advances in the pharmacy teaching-learning methodologies. Hence, I am presenting this reference book as a guide to all pharmacy professionals (students, teachers, pharmacists and governing body). This book provides a detailed overview on teaching philosophy, pharmacy professionalism, basics and innovations associated with the pharmacy teaching-learning methodologies, traditional and modern teaching-learning media/aids and student's performance evaluation. I am confident that this book will update the student's, teacher's, pharmacist's and governing body's knowledge and serve as a guide to improve the quality of teaching-learning.

"Teacher is the one who never ceases to learn"

—S Radhakrishnan

In addition to the overview on the pharmacy teaching-learning methods, this book also provide basic knowledge on how to conduct 'good' educational research, build research skills in students, write a good manuscript/paper, guide students, write a good thesis/dissertation and transform a thesis to manuscript. I am sure that the research basics provided in this book will certainly guide students, trainee and faculty to perform their roles (conducting good educational research, building basic research skills, effective guiding/mentoring students, writing good manuscript and thesis and transforming a thesis to manuscript).

"Without books, history is silent, literature dumb, science crippled, thought and speculation at a standstill"

—Barbara W. Tuchman

Kashappa Goud H. Desai

M. Pharm., Ph. D

ACKNOWLEDGEMENTS

In most of mankind gratitude is merely a secret hope for greater favors.

—Duc de la Rochefoucauld

I am indebted to Mrs. Shobha Churi, JSS College of Pharmacy, Mysore, India, for writing five chapters on important aspects. Some of the chapters incorporate recent advancements in teaching-learning and has helped to increase the scope of the book.

I am also deeply indebted to Dr. Manjunatha B, Associate Professor, Department of Forensic Medicine, JSS Medical College, Mysore, India, for his valuable help, encouragement and comments.

Last but not least, I am grateful to publishers Anmol Publications Pvt. Ltd., New Delhi, India, for taking up this project and publishing the book in time for the benefit of all pharmacy professionals.

Kashappa Goud H. Desai

M. Pharm., Ph. D

LIST OF CONTRIBUTORS

Kashappa Goud H. Desai, M. Pharm., Ph. D
Department Pharmaceutical Sciences
College of Pharmacy,
University of Michigan, Ann Arbor,
Michigan, USA

Shobha Churi, M. Pharm
Department of Pharmacy Practice
JSS College of Pharmacy
SS Nagar, Mysore, India

Section I

TEACHING-LEARNING

Chapter 1
TEACHING PHILOSOPHY

Kashappa Goud H. Desai

"Your time is limited, but your imagination is not"

—Van Crouch

"Plan your work, work your plan"

—Patrick L. Knueven

Philosophy of teaching is a statement articulated by a faculty concerning his perception and description of teaching-learning methods and justification to the proposed teaching-learning methods.

INTRODUCTION

Giving an effective lecture requires a good planning of the chapter contents and delivery modalities. Faculty's responsibilities do not end at the completion of assigned classes. In fact, effective teaching is one of the key components of teaching philosophy. To be a scholarly activity, teaching should be purposeful, reflective, documented, and shared in an evaluative forum. Therefore, before starting the teaching career, articulating a well-defined statement of teaching philosophy is essential to create and maintain a campus culture supportive of teaching. Individual teaching philosophy provides the foundation to clarify goals, guide behavior, seed scholarly dialogue on teaching and organize evaluation. This activity ultimately promotes professional and personal growth. Statements of teaching philosophy function both personally and publicly.

Overseas academic institutions ask faculty and graduate teaching assistants to articulate their philosophy of teaching. This requirement may be in conjunction with the submission of a teaching philosophy statement for seeking academic positions or as a regular component of the portfolio or dossier for promotion and tenure. A statement of teaching philosophy is also requested of candidates for teaching awards or grant applications. Indian academic institutions need to adopt and implement this beneficial criterion while handling above mentioned academic processes. This transformation (process of identifying a personal philosophy of teaching and continuously examining, testifying, and verifying this philosophy through teaching) can change the teaching behaviors and ultimately promote professional, personal, and institutional growth.

ROLE OF STATEMENT OF TEACHING PHILOSOPHY

Teaching is a scholarly activity and serves many purposes. The overlapping contexts where statements of teaching philosophy might function are: *1*) for teaching faculty, 2) for administrators, and *3*) for students.

For Teaching Faculty

1) Basically, a statement of teaching philosophy reveals one's identity as a teacher while also providing a focus or theme for teaching activities.
2) A statement of teaching philosophy describes the role of teaching in relation to other professional responsibilities. The statement can help teaching faculty to monitor their commitments and integrate their professional responsibilities of teaching, research and service.
3) It is a matter to share with colleagues. Then, the statement can serve as an occasion for professional dialogue, growth and development.
4) Teaching philosophy with a clear vision provides stability, continuity and long-term guidance to

teaching faculty. For example, due to their various responsibilities (i.e., teaching, research and service), teaching faculty easily become overwhelmed and tempted just to get through each class. A well-defined philosophy can help them remain focused on their teaching goals and to appreciate the personal and professional rewards of teaching. When faculty perceive clearly what they teach and why, they may also feel more confident about future change due to curriculum development or revision.

5) Articulating a statement of teaching philosophy demonstrates the desire to grow as a professional teacher. The commitment to learning leads him or her to clarify and document values and vision at any given moment. Through professional and personal growth, what is expressed in the statement likely evolves and changes throughout one's career. Teaching faculty who periodically review and update their statements of teaching philosophies make exemplary role models as life-long learners for students and others with whom they interact.

For Administrators

Every academic institution/university has its own mission to accomplish. As the academic scenario evolve constantly and becomes challenging, it becomes necessary for all the teaching faculty and administrators to work collectively to accomplish the institutional/university's mission. The administrators should ask the teaching faculty to match or link their teaching ideologies/goals to the institutional or university's mission statement. To do so, teaching faculty need to answer couple of questions in their statement of teaching philosophy. The questions are: *1*) why are you here at this campus and *2*) why is your presence good for you and good for this institution/university? While achieving their individual ambitions, values, philosophies, attitudes and ethical beliefs, the teaching faculty help shape the institution/university. Administrators should make the statements of teaching philosophy mandatory and this can reflect an institution's/university's focus on the importance of good teaching. It is the responsibility of institutional administrators to guide the teaching faculty's professional growth and achievement. Administrators can provide better support and reward the efforts of teaching faculty in implementing and achieving the components of their teaching philosophies. This can stimulate innovation among faculty members.

When an institution or university creates and maintains a campus culture supportive of teaching, the administrators needs to evaluate teacher's instruction. This is a challenging task as administrators need to answer the question, "how does one recognize achievement when strengths and styles differ?" It can be performed by going through the components of individual teaching philosophy. Using the statement of teaching philosophy, importance given to the academic freedom and responsibility needs to be evaluated. Commitment to maintaining these characteristics, through an evaluative process that tempts faculty towards standardization of teaching evaluation, requires flexibility and time of administrators. An administration learns about teaching in its campus from reading the statements of its teaching faculty. Such knowledge can be used in responding to changing needs and expectations of students and faculty. Hence, the content of the philosophy statements can influence an administration as it pursues its educational mission.

For Students

Teaching faculty articulates their teaching philosophies and shares it with the students. To achieve the goals, faculty adopts conventional and novel teaching-learning methods. Students should understand the principle and purpose of the teaching philosophy. Students can understand these two aspects through the syllabi, assignments, approaches to teaching-learning, classroom environment, and student-teacher relationships. Once the students understand that they are more benefited by the teaching philosophy, they will be self-motivated and involve productively in teaching-learning methods. Further, students will come to know how to learn and succeed in the course. The goal of sharing a statement of teaching philosophy is to respect and support students by being explicit.

COMPONENTS OF A STATEMENT OF TEACHING PHILOSOPHY

Faculty or an individual wanting to write a statement of teaching philosophy needs to know what to include in their statement. Designing and expression of a teaching philosophy starts with the imagination of teaching. Reading about teaching, watching to what others teach and listening to what other say will help to articulate the statement. Importantly, it is necessary to think beyond what one knows about teaching-learning. Faculty or an individual willing to articulate a statement should stimulate his/her brain to get various innovative ideologies about teaching-learning. Statement of teaching philosophy is very personal by nature, there are no required contents or set skeleton for inclusion and execution. Therefore, it is up to individual to decide what to include in their own statement. However, there are some dimensions (see below) that fulfill the purpose of such statements.

1) **Integration of responsibilities:** Institution or university assigns teaching, research, and service responsibilities to faculty. These three key responsibilities fragment faculty's activity and thinking into three or more channels. As a result, the faculty may prioritize one area and relatively ignore the others. For effective teaching, the concept of these three missions should be melded together and expressed in teaching. It may not be possible when the faculty ignores one of these responsibilities. Faculty should explicitly describe what they do in

carrying out/integrating these three missions and consequent benefits in their statements of teaching philosophy. In addition, it is also important how faculty visualize the institutional or university's mission. Instead of describing themselves as supporting the institutional or university's mission, it is better to present themselves as uniquely contributing to the institutional or university mission in the statement.

2) **Expertise:** Every faculty is an expert in one chosen field of teaching and research. Students perceive effective teachers as one who have knowledge of the subject matter. Therefore, the statement of teaching philosophy should contain one's unique modes by which he/she teach their special knowledge or expertise to the students. Further, they should also mention about their ability to communicate that knowledge clearly and enthusiastically. Importantly, the statement should describe expertise and modes of teaching-learning in the context of a discipline in the institution or university.

3) **Relationships:** Healthy teacher-students relationship is essential to successful teaching. Such a healthy relationship will create the desired teaching and learning environment. Therefore, every faculty should describe modes by which he/she create and maintain the positive relationship with the students. In particular, the ways the faculty adopts to know the students and build rapport with the students. In addition, the teaching-learning environment can be enhanced when a faculty works effectively with other personnel. Thus, issues of effective collaboration could also be explored in a statement of teaching philosophy.

4) **Learning environment:** Once the classrooms are assigned, a faculty can do additional work to create

an environment favorable to teaching-learning. For example, modifications to the built environment (e.g., rearranging chairs and using technology), social environment (e.g., using collaborative or co-operative teaching strategies), psychological environment (e.g., defining expectations) and physical boundaries of the classrooms (e.g., adding e-mail and out-of-class meetings to the course structure). These and any other novel ideas can be included in a purposeful manner in the statement of teaching philosophy.

5) **Methods, strategies and innovation:** There are numerous teaching-learning methods, strategies and tips. A faculty can include well-tested and novel approaches in the statement. Importantly, a faculty should answer why, what and how his/her teaching-learning is done. Further, how teaching strategies match one's philosophical assumptions about learning and the objectives of teaching.

6) **Outcome:** The objectives of teaching is to communicate effectively with the students about succeeding in a course and making a difference in their lives, receive and maintain accreditation, and meet expectations of growth and change. In the statement of teaching philosophy, faculty should express how the previous efforts have produced anticipated outcomes and their view of the intended outcomes of teaching. For example, faculty should express what students have gained and will gain (e.g., thinking skills, attitudes, values, technical skills, etc.) from teaching-learning courses.

RECOMMENDATIONS TO THE MANAGEMENT

The process of articulation, implementation and evaluation of teaching philosophy will make the faculty to compare themselves between theoretical and actual self. The management should facilitate the process to allow a personal reflection and variety of outcomes. Every institution or universitv has its own protocol for faculty review, retention, promotion and merit pay. However, following are the recommendations that can be adapted for promoting teacher's efficiency. These recommendations can guide the management as they work with the faculty.

- The management (administrators and institutional/ university leaders) needs to build a supportive network and opinion for discussion on statements of teaching philosophy, teaching portfolios and institutional review of teaching.
- The management needs to develop a supportive framework for faculty discussions of teaching performance, evaluation and excellence. In particular, the administration needs to allow each department to set criteria of evaluation and rewards/promotions for varied/novel modes of teaching-learning.
- Develop an environment in which the faculty can lead the teaching discussions by asking a lot of probing questions and supporting a variety of perspectives.
- Needs to emphasize on "why do the teachers teach in the ways they do"?
- Statement of teaching philosophy varies from person to person and so the growth of the faculty. Therefore, let the context of the statement of teaching philosophy determine its content, format and presentation.
- The management needs to motivate and encourage the faculty to define themselves and their roles in relation to the institution/university mission.
- A faculty integrates teaching, research and service responsibilities. Therefore, prompt commitment to a teaching philosophy and guidance is required from the management.

REFERENCES

1. Chism NVN. 1998. Developing a philosophy of teaching statement. Essays on Teaching Excellence. Professional and organizational development network in higher education 9:1-2.
2. Goodyear GE. Allchin D. 1998. Statement of teaching philosophy. To improve the academy17:103-22. New Forums Press, Stillwater, OK.
3. Rodriguez-Farrar HB. 1997. The teaching portfolio: A handbook for faculty, teaching assistants and teaching fellows (2nd Ed.). Brown University, Harriet sheridan center for teaching and learning.
4. Bernoff RA. 1992. Effective teaching techniques: A workshop. Paper presented at the national conference on successful college teaching and administration. Orlando, Florida.
5. Grasha AF. 1996. Teaching with style: A practical guide to enhancing learning by understanding teaching and learning styles. Alliance Publishers, Pittsburgh, PA.

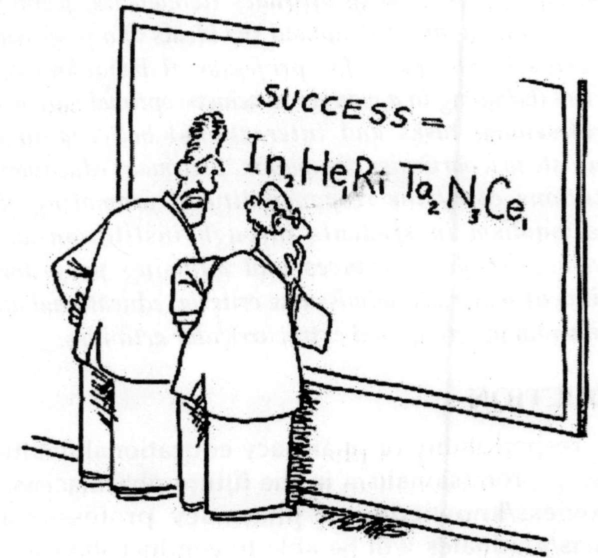

"Doctor, I believe you've found the formula for success."

Chapter 2
PHARMACY PROFESSIONALISM

Kashappa Goud H. Desai

"We may never have the opportunity to do great things in a great way, but we all have the chance to do small things in a great way"

Professionalism is a set of attitudes (tendencies, feelings, emotions or thoughts that uphold the ideals of a profession and serves as the basis for professional behavior) and behaviors (behaving in a manner to achieve optimal outcomes in professional tasks and interactions) believed to be appropriate to a particular occupation. Pharmacy educational institutions carry the responsibility of promoting the professionalism in students through institution-wide initiatives, student services and advising programs, recruitment materials, admissions criteria, educational and experimental programs and extracurricular activities.

INTRODUCTION

The basic responsibility of pharmacy educational institutions is to develop professionalism in the future pharmacists. With the awareness/knowledge of pharmacy professionalism, pharmacists/graduates will be able to conduct themselves in a better manner, perform adequate pharmaceutical care and can provide better service to humanity. Fulfilling these responsibilities by future pharmacists/graduates can promote the status of pharmacy profession to a new level. Therefore, the pharmacy institutions need to focus on this vital concern and build the professionalism in their students.

Professionalism is a set of attitudes (tendencies, feelings, emotions or thoughts that uphold the ideals of a profession and serves as the basis for professional behavior) and behaviors (behaving in a manner to achieve optimal outcomes in professional tasks and interactions) believed to be appropriate to a particular occupation or the active demonstration of the traits of a professional constitute. In other words, a manner that is created through a combination of behaviors, including courtesy and politeness when dealing with patients, peers and other health care professionals. Pharmacists should consistently display respect for others and maintain appropriate boundaries of privacy and discretion.

PHARMACY PROFESSIONAL ATTITUDES AND BEHAVIORS (COMPONENTS OF PHARMACY PROFESSIONALISM)

Professional attitudes and their corresponding behaviors are listed in Table 2.1. These attitudes and behaviors are appropriate for students as well as teachers. Pharmacy institutions need to foster these attitudes and behaviors in the academic environment.

Table 2.1

Professional attitudes and corresponding behaviors for pharmacy students and teachers[a]

Attitude	Behavior
Accountability	Takes responsibility for actions
Caring	Volunteering, acts of service
Desire for self-improvement	Continued learning, self-instruction
Diversity	Fair treatment of all people regardless of demographic characteristics

Honesty	Behaviors that demonstrate honesty and trustworthiness
Open-minded	Increased receptiveness to new ideas
Respect	Dresses appropriately, punctual, maintains confidentiality
Responsibility to learn	Comes to class prepared, actively participates in class activities such as discussion
Team player	Engages in constructive peer assessment, accepts and applies constructive critique
Values new experiences	Desire to seek out and take on new challenges

[a]Submitted by participants in the 2000 American Association of College of Pharmacy (AACP) Teacher's Seminar on Developing Professional Attitudes and Behaviors.

PROMOTING PROFESSIONALISM (ATTITUDES AND BEHAVIORS) IN THE ACADEMIC ENVIRONMENT

Following are some ideas and examples of how pharmacy educational institutions can promote professional attitudes and behaviors in their academic program.

1) **Institution-wide initiatives:** Include professional attitudes and behavioral components in the institutional mission statement. Institutions need to demonstrate or explain or conduct role-play about effective interpersonal and interprofessional interactions, self-assessment, self-directed learning and professional and social responsibility.

2) **Student services and advising programs:** Student services and student's advisors should help students to develop professional attitudes, ethics and behaviors. Institutions need to give provision for these activities.

3) **Recruitment:** Institutions need to develop recruitment materials and processes in such a way that they demonstrate professionalism of the academic programs and profession. While recruiting students,

emphasize on the professional roles of students and pharmacists. For example, taking a statement on 'pharmacy student's professionalism' along with recruiting materials.

4) **Admissions:** Institutional admissions criteria, policies and procedures are giving significant consideration to the student's academic accomplishments. Other factors such as motivation, industry and communication capabilities should also be considered while admitting the students. With these additional characteristics, students will become a life-long learner and an effective professional.

5) **Educational program:** Institutions need to organize an orientation program for new students. In this orientation program, discuss the roles and responsibilities of pharmacists including the oath of a pharmacist and code of ethics for pharmacists. This is an excellent opportunity to begin and develop professionalism among students.

6) **Experimental programs:** The behaviors that students may demonstrate in the practice are likely to be displayed by them during their experimental rotations. Therefore, educators should employ some sort of behavioral evaluation of students while they are participating in experimental rotations.

7) **Extracurricular activities:** Educators should actively encourage students to involve in various professional organizations, serve as role models and attend the national, state and local meetings. In addition, educators should also put organized efforts to broaden the horizons of students (scientific inquiry, scholarly concern for the profession and post-graduate education and training through guest lecturers and participation in curricular and extracurricular activities).

MEASUREMENT OF PHARMACY PROFESSIONALISM

Valid and reliable instruments are necessary to measure student's professionalism. Following are ways to collect attitudinal and behavioral data.

Attitudinal data collection: Student 'attitude' data can be traditionally collected via self-administered questionnaires to determine attitudes toward many different referents such as the profession of pharmacy, pharmacy curricula, professional commitment and the provision of pharmaceutical care. Briefly, a questionnaire comprising numerous questions about the attitudes should be prepared. Then, the students should be asked to indicate the extent to which they agree or disagree with each of the questions using a five-point Likert-type scale ranging from strongly disagree to strongly agree (1 = strongly disagree, 2 = disagree, 3 = neutral, 4 = agree, and 5 = strongly agree). Participation in the study needs to be voluntary and the identity of the participants should be blinded to the investigators. Finally, calculate the required statistical data. Scores of negatively worded items should be reversed so that higher scores reflect more positive attitudes.

Behavioral data collection: Behavioral data on students can be collected in two ways: *a*) students self-report (how they have behaved in certain situations or how they predict they would behave in certain situations and *b*) observation by others. Student self-report data can be collected through questionnaires or portfolios. Among the two options, observation by the teachers is the most reliable data sources. Behavioral assessment by teachers can be performed using the behavioral professionalism assessment form/ questionnaire. Briefly, a questionnaire comprising numerous questions that can assess student's behavioral skills (see below) should be prepared.

1) Reliable and dependable (can be counted on to fulfill responsibilities and meet expectations).

2) Practices personal hygiene (maintains personal health and grooming habits acceptable to practice setting).

3) Produces quality work (tasks and assignments are complete, accurate and meet their respective objectives).

4) Empathetic (demonstrates appreciation of other's positions, attempts to identify with other's perspectives and consideration towards others).

5) Behaves in an ethical manner (acts in the best interest of others).

6) Communicates articulately (clearly communicates thoughts, uses appropriate terminology and vocabulary for intended audience).

7) Punctual (arrives to class and meetings early or on time, meets deadlines for completion of tasks and responsibilities).

8) Uses time efficiently (allocates and utilizes appropriate amounts of time to fulfill responsibilities and utilizes other's time wisely).

9) Self-directed in undertaking tasks (after initial instruction of tasks/assignments/responsibilities, initiates activities to complete them, self-motivated, functions independently).

10) Handles stress (remains clam, levelheaded and composed in critical, stressful and difficult situations).

11) Respectful (demonstrates regard for self, standardized patients, peers, faculty, staff and institution property).

12) Communicates using appropriate body language (utilizes gestures and mannerisms that enhance formal and informal communication).

13) Demonstrates accountability (holds oneself liable for tasks/ duties/responsibilities that he/she is responsible and does not blame others for mistakes or mishaps, nor avoids responsibilities).

14) Prioritizes responsibilities effectively (organizes and approaches multiple tasks and assignments in a manner to produce desired outcomes).
15) Accepts and applies constructive criticism (responds openly and positively to feedback, modifies behavior if necessary).
16) Puts other's needs above his/her own (demonstrates an attitude of service by taking the necessary time and actions to help others, gives of oneself to benefit others).
17) Nonjudgmental (demonstrates an attitude of open-mindedness towards others and situations and does not 'stereotype' others or prejudge situations).
18) Communicates assertively (actively and appropriately engages in dialogue or discussion, not afraid to provide his/her viewpoint).
19) An active learner (seeks knowledge, asks questions, searches for information, takes responsibility for own learning).
20) Cooperative (non-argumentative, willing and helpful).
21) Diplomatic (fair and tactful in all dealings with standardized patients, peers, faculty and staff).
22) Follows through with responsibilities (if task is left incomplete or problem is not resolved, student seeks aid).
23) Wears appropriate attire (adheres to dress code as outlined in the course syllabus).
24) Demonstrates confidence (acts and communicates in a self-assured manner, yet with modesty and humility).
25) Demonstrates a desire to exceed expectations (goes 'above and beyond the call of duty', attempts to

exceed minimal standards and requirements for tasks/ assignments/responsibilities).

Then, the teachers should indicate the extent to which they agree or disagree with each of the skills using a five-point Likert-type scale ranging from strongly disagree to strongly agree (1 = strongly disagree, 2 = disagree, 3 = neutral, 4 = agree, and 5 = strongly agree). Finally, calculate the required statistical data.

REFERENCES

1. Bucher R, Stelling J. 1977. Becoming professional (1st ed). Sage publications, Beverly Hills, CA, USA.
2. Montague JB. 1968. Pharmacy and the concept of professionalism. Journal of American Pharmaceutical Association NS8:228-230.
3. Chalmers RK. 1997. Contemporary issues: Professionalism in pharmacy. Tomorrow's Pharmacist 3:10-12.
4. American Board of Internal Medicine (ABIM). 1995. Project professionalism. ABIM committee on evaluation of clinical competence, Philadelphia, PA, USA.
5. APhA-ASP/AACP-COD. 2000. Task force on professionalism. White paper on pharmacy student professionalism. Journal of American Pharmaceutical Association 40:96-102.
6. Civility/professionalism. 2000. 101st AACP Annual Meeting, July 8, San Diego, California, USA.

Chapter 3
TEACHING-LEARNING METHODS

Kashappa Goud H. Desai

"Education is not the amount of information that is put into your brain and runs there, undigested, all your life. We must have life-building, man-making, character-building, assimilating fine ideas and making them your life and character, you have more education than any man who has got by heart a whole library"

—Swami Vivekananda

"And without method there is neither organization nor construction"

—Bulwer

CLASSIFICATION/TYPES OF TEACHING-LEARNING METHODS

A) Large group methods

1) Traditional lecture
2) Interactive lecture
3) Panel discussion
4) Case based teaching-learning method
5) Symposium

B) Small group methods

1) Problem based teaching-learning method
2) Group discussion

3) Seminar
4) Tutorial
5) Demonstration
6) Practicals/field work
7) Role play
8) Workshop

C) Advanced (information and communication technology-based) teaching-learning methods

1) Teaching-learning with audio-video tape
2) Computer assisted teaching-learning method
3) Web based teaching-learning method
4) Online teaching-learning method
5) Mobile teaching-learning method
6) Pharmacy informatics
7) Distance learning

D) Individual methods

1) Reading
2) Project work
3) Assignment
4) Self-study

In the forthcoming segment of the book, only the important teaching-learning methods are discussed. These include: *1*) interactive lecture, *2*) problem based teaching-learning, *3*) case based teaching-learning, *4*) computer assisted teaching-learning, *5*) Web based teaching-learning, *6*) online teaching-learning, *7*) mobile teaching-learning and *8*) pharmacy informatics methods.

Chapter 4
INTERACTIVE LECTURE—A BETTER APPROACH AND WAYS TO PERFORM

Kashappa Goud H. Desai

"Students hear and they may forget; they see and they remember; they interact and they understand"

Interactive lecture is a modified version of traditional lecture in which numerous learning enhancement features (two-way interaction, communication, and questioning, small group and problem solving activities, and supporting media) are incorporated and performed orally to teach the particular subject information to the students by a teacher.

INTRODUCTION

Centuries ago, the lecture was formerly started as a teaching process. The teaching process began with a literal reading of important passages from the text by the master, followed by the master's interpretation of the text. Students were expected to sit, listen and take notes. Thereafter, with little or no modifications, the traditional lecture is being commonly used as a method of teaching in the institutions/universities. The reasons for preferring the traditional lecture method are: *a*) most of us were taught by this method, *b*) it appears easy to prepare and present, and *c*) the method is accepted by students and peers. The strengths of traditional lecture method are given below.

Strengths of Traditional Lecture Method

1) Lecture method presents factual material in direct and logical manner
2) This method contains experience which inspires the students
3) It stimulates students thinking to open discussion
4) It is useful for teaching large groups

However, traditional lecture can lead to ineffective teaching if all the classroom teaching features are not adopted. The major limitation of the lecture method is the lack of interaction between teacher and students. Various classroom modifications need to be adopted to transform the traditional lecture into an interactive lecture (see Table 4.1).

WAYS TO PERFORM INTERACTIVE LECTURE

It is not a simple job for the teachers to transform the traditional lecture into an interactive lecture. The manner of speaking and mode of lecture delivery immeasurably influence student's attentiveness and learning. Further, voice, gesture, movement, facial expression, and eye contact will either complement or detract from the content while teaching. Person may be new to the lecture format or has spent several years presenting lectures, teacher needs to perform three key functions to transform the traditional lecture into an interactive lecture. Planning, delivery and evaluation are the three key characteristics of an interactive lecture. Further, effective classroom communication and presentation skills also play important roles while achieving the goal (interactive teaching-learning).

1) Planning of Interactive Lecture

Planning of interactive lecture begins by deciding the outcome(s) of the lecture in advance. Planning of interactive lecture can be done by completing the following tasks: planning of lecture contents, planning the delivery of lecture contents, considering the lecture logistics (length, number of students, and size and shape of the lecture room), media equipment and preparation of lecture notes.

Table 4.1.

Features of traditional and interactive lecture methods

Feature	Traditional Lecture	Interactive Lecture
Interaction	100% teacher's talk, with limited or no interaction	Teacher-students
Communication	One-way	Two-way
Questioning	Few if any (teacher or student)	Teacher-student questions
Responsibility	Students depends on teacher for all information	Shared for active learning
Student activities	No	Small group, problem solving
Supporting media	No	Variety of supporting media
Note taking	Extensive	Limited (student have copies of lecture notes)

A) Planning of lecture contents: The contents of lecture can be sub-divided and prepared as given below.

a) Purpose and objective of the lecture: In this section, teachers should decide about the purpose and objective of the lecture. The basic purpose of the lecture is to convey/transfer the information from teacher to the students. However, the purpose (non-measurable term) clarifies what students will learn during the lecture. In contrast, objective is precise and measurable term which describes what student will learn by attending the lecture. Depending on the requirement, teacher can consider purpose, objective or both while planning the interactive lecture. Following is an example of a lecture topic with both a purpose statement and objective.

Lecture topic: Development of tablets

Purpose: The purpose of this lecture is to acquaint the students with tablets and shape of the tablets, ingredients of tablets, methods of preparation of tablets, and role of tablets.

Objective: After completion of lecture, students shall be able to describe the advantages of various kinds of tablets, role of each ingredient of the tablets, principles and procedure of methods of preparation of tablets, and applications of each class of tablets.

b) ***Key points***: Students will lose sight of the main ideas when a teacher gives too many details. Therefore, it is necessary to strike a balance between depth and breadth of coverage. This can be done by writing and presenting the key points of the lecture while teaching.

c) ***Introduction, body and summary of the lecture***: The planned introduction should be able to capture the interest and attention of the students. Introduction can also make students aware of the teacher's expectations and encourage a positive learning environment. A good introduction is critical to the success of a lecture. Secondly, a focused body of the lecture should be able to examine major concepts of lecture. Lastly, a resounding summary should connect and bring closure to the concepts covered.

B) Planning the delivery of lecture contents: Once a teacher determines the goals (what student will learn) of a lecture and organizes the lecture contents, the next step is to plan how best those contents can be presented or delivered in a classroom. The three main parts of a lecture are introduction, body, and summary. Therefore, a teacher needs to plan how well an introduction, body, and summary can be delivered to the students.

a) ***Planning of a catchy introduction***: The objective of introduction is to capture the interest and attention of the students. Try some of the following strategies to achieve it.

- Review the objective(s) of lecture.
- Ask various questions (related to the lecture topic) to the students.
- Ask students to show their hands as a response to the questions.
- Use an interesting or famous quotation.
- Relate the topic to previously covered content.
- Use a case study or problem-solving activity.
- Use a videotape or other media.
- Show an appropriate cartoon with the overhead or slide projector.
- Make a provocative statement to encourage discussion.
- Give a demonstration.
- Use a game or role play.
- Relate the topic to future work experiences.
- Share a personal experience.
- Relate the topic to a real-life experience.

b) ***Balancing the lecture (body of lecture)***: Once the attention of the students has been captured with an interesting introduction, teacher should make a smooth transition into the body of the lecture. In this section, a teacher needs to plan how the body (core information to be transferred to the students) of the lecture will be delivered to the students. Break the presentation for about 3-5 minute exercises that require students to interact with the lecture content, their notes and each other (for example, brainstorming, discussions, problem-solving activities, case studies and games). This makes the lecture more interactive. These active-learning processes also stimulate students for group discussion.

c) ***Planning the delivery of lecture summary***: The teacher should conclude the lecture by delivering the summary which should draw together critical information presented. The summary should also ensure that students leave the lecture with a clear understanding of the information. Importantly, the summary should be brief and address only key points. Following are the some strategies which can be used to summarize a lecture.

- Ask the students if they have questions. This gives students an opportunity to clarify their understanding of the content.
- Ask questions to the students. Several questions which focus on the key points of the lecture may be used to summarize.
- Use a transparency, slide or flipchart to review the summary points.

C) **Considering the logistics of lecture:** In this section, teacher should decide/know about the length of the lecture, number of students, size and shape of the lecture room and media equipment.

a) ***Length:*** Generally, the length of traditional lecture varies from 30-45 minutes including questioning if any. The length of interactive lecture should not be more than 60 minutes without a break, based on the teacher's experience.

b) ***Number of students:*** The number of students attending the class will decide the mode of presentation of an interactive lecture. By knowing the group size, use of questions, amount of interaction, selection and use of media (e.g., overhead transparencies, slides, computer-based projections, video, audio etc.) and use of small group activities (e.g., case studies, role plays and problem-solving exercises) can be determined. For example, Table 4.2 shows the estimates of how the number of students can have an impact on the use of questioning, the most common form of interaction while lecturing.

Table 4.2

Effect of student's group size on the method of questioning

Number of Students	Method of Questioning
1-30	Questioning is two-way (teacher-student). Students discuss lecture doubts with teacher and among themselves
31-50	Questioning is two-way (teacher-student). But, limited discussion among the students
51-100	Teacher asks questions, and only a small number of the students answer them. Students ask some questions. Students are able to discuss doubts only with other students seated near them. There is little or no feedback to the teacher
>100	Teacher asks questions, and students raise their hands to either agree or disagree. There will be very few comments or questions from the students. Students are able to discuss content only with other students seated near them. There is little or no feedback to the teacher.

c) ***Size and shape of the room***: Planning and delivery of the interactive lecture is also influenced by the size and shape of the lecture room. Following are some examples.

- A room with tables arranged in a U-shape and chairs for 20 students is good for small group's interactive lectures.

- A large room with 100 chairs arranged in a theater-mode with an aisle down the middle makes it possible for the lecturer to move up and down the aisle to interact with students (large group interactive lecture).

D) Media equipment: The lecture hall should be able to accommodate the use of slides, overhead transparencies, video and computer based projections. A teacher needs to use variety of media to teach the students effectively.

E) Preparation of lecture notes: Many teachers ignore the importance of lecture notes. Many times, teachers think that they know, can remember and deliver the lecture contents effectively without the support of lecture notes. However, this will lead to unsatisfactory experience for both the teacher and students. Therefore, teachers should prepare the lecture notes to serve as a script of set of clues to follow during the interactive lecture. Lecture notes can be prepared in the form of key words, phrases, and other reminders (e.g., audiovisual clues, questions, examples, notes for activities) but organized into an outline format. Following are the roles of the lecture notes.

- Lecture notes helps teacher to stay on topic and prevent getting lost.
- These notes help to cover the key points and avoid forgetting any parts of the lecture.
- These notes help to glance at a specific point and quickly return attention to the students.
- Lecture notes allow the teacher to relax and focus on delivery instead of worrying about what point to make next.

2) Delivery of Interactive Lecture

The lecture delivery is the most exciting and rewarding job for the teachers. Once the planning of the lecture (goals (what needs to be taught and modes of teaching) and notes of the interactive lecture) is completed, it is necessary to know the ways for effective delivery of lecture contents. An effective teacher is one who helps students to reach the learning objectives. This job can be done by making the dynamic delivery using variety of teaching-learning methods and maintaining the student's interest with an excitement. When teacher and students interact, discuss, question and work together, it can be called as an interactive/effective lecture. To create an active teaching-learning environment in the classroom, teachers should adopt the suggested techniques (see below) for questioning the students and presenting the lecture. In addition, ways to handle the presentation anxiety are also given below.

a) **Questioning techniques:** By asking the questions to the students and stimulating the students to raise the questions, a teacher can create an interactive environment in the classroom and maintain the student's attention throughout the class. Questions can be asked while introducing the lecture, stimulating the students and summarizing the lecture. Following are some suggestions for teachers on how to conduct questioning.

   - Check student understanding about the key aspects of the lecture by asking various questions. Verify the student's responses by providing the correct answer. Show answer(s) on the board or overhead display or flipchart etc. Guide the incorrect answers by asking a guiding question, explaining the missing idea and then allow student to answer, and describing what student is doing wrong.

   - Method of asking the question: First ask at a recall level, and then gradually increase to more complex levels (comprehension, analysis, synthesis, application and evaluation).

- Teacher needs to ask questions to all the students. Stimulate students to volunteer in questioning. Some students may not involve in a questioning. Therefore, teacher must guard against some students dominating the discussion.
- Choose a specific question and ask it to a specific student. If the group size is relatively small, this technique can be used to involve more of the students.
- Recognize each student and use student's name while performing the classroom activities (questioning, group discussion, and problem solving activities). This will motivate the students.
- Whenever students respond or react to a particular question or interact in the learning activities, praise or give positive support to the students for their response. This attitude will create a very positive environment and encourage other students to enter into the learning activities.
- Whenever a student asks a question, repeat the question and answer to ensure that all students hear the conversation/discussion.
- Whenever a student asks a question, the teacher can answer the question directly, respond by asking the student a different, related question or offer the question to the other students.

b) **Presentation techniques:** The teachers should use variety of presentation techniques to engage students in learning activities, maintain their interest, and avoid repetitive lecturing style. Following are some techniques that can be used to make the lecture more interactive and effective.

- Arrive at class a few minutes early and chat with students about topics other than your upcoming lecture.

- While lecturing, use the lecture notes (key words, phrases, or reminders) appropriately.
- Using one or more strategies mentioned in the planning section (planning of various strategies for a catchy introduction), give a catchy introduction. The introduction should capture the attention and interest of the students.
- Interact and communicate with each student. The teacher should relate the subject matter to the students while teaching.
- Using the appropriate inter-connecting sentence, make the smooth transitions between parts of the lecture (introduction, body and summary).
- Make and maintain the eye contact with students. This gives the teacher feedback on student's understanding about concepts and helps to communicate back with the students.
- Show the enthusiasm while lecturing. Varying the speech, changing the eye movement (raise eyebrows; open eyes wide), moving around the room, showing high degree of energy/vitality, smiling, facial expression, and being supportive are some examples of showing enthusiasm.
- Use variety in the voice. Students sitting in the back of the room should hear the volume clearly. Use microphone if necessary. Change the volume from forceful to soft. Change speed and tempo of the speech.
- Speak to the students, not to the board, flip-chart, or overhead
- Avoid using the slang or repetitive words/phrases (e.g., "um", "er", "you know", "okay" "uhhh").
- Use audiovisuals (e. g., tape, handouts, flipchart, and overhead projector, liquid crystal display) to increase the understanding and impact.

- Ask a number of questions to students and encourage them to ask questions. Give positive feedback for student's questions.
- Refer or use student's name as often as possible.
- Share or display a positive use of humor.
- Give brief and powerful summary of the lecture.

c) Ways to handle presentation anxiety

- Take a light meal before the lecture. Eating a big meal will full stomach and make you drowsy. It will be difficult to move around the room with energy.
- Go for a short walk just before the lecture.
- Reach the classroom early and make sure that everything (additional arrangements, lighting, and media equipment) is ready before the first student arrives.
- Decide where the lecture notes will be placed (e.g., on a lectern, desk, table) when they are not being held.
- Take a look over the lecture notes.
- Take a few deep breaths to relax before beginning the lecture.
- Drink a glass of water during the lecture.

3) Evaluation of Interactive Lecture

Effective planning and delivery of interactive lecture do not instantly mean that students grasped the key concepts of the lecture. Once the interactive lecture is completed, the following questions should arise in a teacher's or evaluator's (higher authority) mind.

- Did the lecture make any difference?
- How effective was the teacher in transferring knowledge to the students?

- Will the information have an impact?
- Did the students enjoy the lecture?
- How can the teacher improve the next lecture?

Therefore, teacher's interactive lecture should be evaluated by an appropriate evaluation technique. However, evaluation questions are easy to ask and often difficult to answer. To seek answers to the above mentioned questions, one of the following evaluation techniques can be adopted.

a) **Student feedback:** Student feedback can be taken in different forms (One-minute note card, open notebook quiz, and periodic surveys).

- ***One-minute note card*:** In the final few minutes of class, ask everyone to write two details on a note card: *1*) one topic, concept, idea, or lesson that they understand clearly from the lecture and *2*) one question that they still have about the lecture. After receiving the cards, review all the cards and find answers to these questions: *1*) do students typically have questions about material you cover at the beginning, middle, or end of your lecture? and 2) do they understand topics more clearly when you engage them into active learning exercises? Accordingly, improve your lecture format.

- ***Open notebook quiz*:** At the end of some interactive lectures, held an unannounced open notebook quiz. Write or post 3-5 questions on the board or overhead transparency or PowerPoint slide. The questions should be such that those cover the important definitions, facts and stimulate critical thinking of the students. This exercise emphasizes the importance of note taking during lectures and gives students a glimpse of the material you consider most important in the day's lesson. The response from the students is'the feedback for the teacher's lecture.

- ***Periodic surveys***: Plan and conduct evaluation of course lectures (content and delivery), readings, assignments, and classroom environment in a detailed (8-12 question) survey. Surveys can be monthly and/or at mid-term, revising questions based on the feedback you seek. This survey asks for student's opinion on course content and delivery, not the student's understanding of the content. Therefore, it should be completed anonymously.

b) **Self-evaluation:** It is a very effective evaluation technique. In this technique, video recording of the interactive lecture is done. Then, a teacher should critique a videotape of his lecture. Analyzing a video allows the teacher to identify positive and negative behaviors, set specific goals for improving the quality of lectures, and improve the presentation skills. Self-analysis can be done alone or with an experienced presenter. In each case, teacher's presentation strengths and areas needing improvement should be evaluated using an interactive lecture skills evaluation form.

c) **Use of an observer:** In this technique, teacher's skills are evaluated by an observer. The observer must be an experienced presenter. The observer should sit in the classroom, watch the interactive lecture, and give the feedback (aspects of lecture that were effective and lecture skills needing improvement) in the interactive lecture skills evaluation form.

REFERENCES

1. Beitz JM. 1994. Dynamics of effective oral presentations: Strategies for nurse educators. AORN Journal 59:1026-1032.
2. Renner P. 1993. The art of teaching adults. Training associates, Vancouver, British Columbia.

3. Vella F. 1992. Medical education: Capitalizing on the lecture method. FASEB Journal 6: 811-812.

4. Price DA and CA Mitchell. 1993. A model for clinical teaching and learning. Medical Education 27:62-68.

5. Silberman ML. 1990. Active Training: A handbook of techniques, designs, case examples, and tips. Lexington Books, New York.

Interactive Lecture Skills Evaluation Form

Instructions: For each teacher, evaluation of interactive lecture can be done 5 times. After every interactive lecture, lecturing skills needing improvement should be noted. Then, set the goals and work hard to improve those skills. By the end of the fifth interactive lecture, teacher should be able to perform all the interactive lecturing skills effectively. Observe the interactive lecture and use the following rating scale to indicate the level of performance of each presentation skills.

A: Teacher is competent at performing this skill and requires no additional practice

B: Teacher can perform this skill but requires additional practice

C: Teacher cannot perform this skill and requires extensive practice

N. O: Skill not observed during this lecture presentation

N. A: Skill not applicable to this lecture presentation

Interactive Lecture Skills Evaluation Form

	Presentation skills	Observations				
		1	2	3	4	5
I	**Preparation skills** Selected lecture methods in advance. Prepared lecture notes in advance. Prepared audiovisuals in advance. Planned effective techniques to introduce the lecture. Arranged room appropriately.					

II	**Verbal skills**					
	Projected voice (changed pitch, tone and volume).					
	Avoided fillers (e.g., "um," "er," "you know," etc.).					
	Used student names.					
	Used familiar terms.					
	Used many examples.					
	Provided praise and reinforcement.					
	Accepted student ideas and suggestions.					
	Used appropriate humor.					
III	**Nonverbal skills**					
	Maintained eye contact.					
	Maintained positive facial expressions.					
	Gestured with hands and arms.					
	Maintained good posture.					
	Moved around the room with energy.					
	Followed lecture notes.					
IV	**Questioning skills**					
	Asked questions at varying levels of difficulty.					
	Asked questions to group.					
	Asked questions to individual students.					
	Involved all students (if possible).					
	Repeated student responses and questions.					
	Provided positive reinforcement.					
V	**Audiovisual skills**					
	Used presentation media correctly.					
VI	**Summarizing skills**					
	Asked for questions.					
	Asked questions.					
	Used media to review main points.					

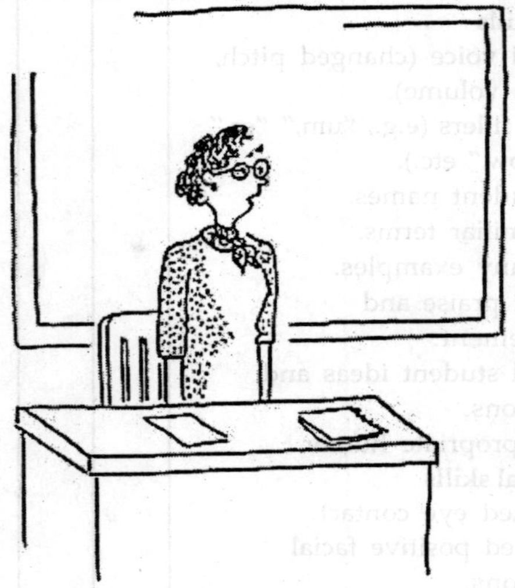

"Before I begin today's lecture, please turn off your cell phones, beepers, and iPods."

Chapter 5

PROBLEM BASED TEACHING-LEARNING: BENEFITS, PROCESS, RESPONSIBILITIES AND INNOVATIONS

Shobha Churi

"PBT-L is not the solution for all problems in education; however, it is a powerful tool for allowing students to actively build collaborative problem solving skills that will be required in the work environment"

—Kanter

Problem based teaching-learning (PBT-L) is a teacher-student discussion based educational methodology in which learning originates from a presented problem. The sequential stages of PBT-L process are understand the presented problem, search the strategies, resolve the problem and evaluate the effectiveness of process. Since it is a student centered active learning process, the success of PBT-L process is mainly governed by the manner in which students perform their responsibilities (self-learning, integrating various disciplines, thinking critically and collaborating and communicating effectively). Traditional PBT-L process has been revolutionized by the introduction of information and communication technologies (ICTs). Computerized and E-mail assisted PBT-L methods have provided more flexible and improvised learning environment.

INTRODUCTION

Traditionally, in pharmacy education, teachers perform didactic, subject oriented and knowledge-based teaching. Although these are essential methods, they do not provide opportunities to learn the pharmacy concepts and processes. In the constantly evolving pharmacy profession, every teacher needs to build problem identification, problem solving and continuing education skills in the students to prepare them to overcome future competencies. Development of teaching methods to build these skills has been a well-recognized objective for improving the quality of pharmacy education. Consistent with this objective, PBT-L has been introduced in the pharmacy education.

Student centered PBT-L methodology utilizes collaborative study of problems in small discussion groups, facilitated by faculty direction that concentrates on group process. The problem engages student's curiosity and drives their learning. Then, students ask themselves numerous critical questions to find solution to the problem. To find appropriate solution and involve actively in the discussion, students perform research on the problem and related concepts, thereby learning the concepts of the subject as well as problem solving skill.

The teacher/tutor acts as a facilitator and resource person to give guidance and advice to students. The discussions in PBT-L force students to use hypothesis driven reasoning, which is more effective than lectures in developing problem solving ability because students must apply scientific knowledge to problems. This method has been widely accepted and enjoyed teaching-learning method by the students and teachers. Unlike the traditional lecture, the PBT-L is a student centered educational approach and create an active learning environment (see Table 5.1 for comparison).

Table 5.1
Traditional lecture vs. PBT-L

Feature	Traditional Lecture	PBT-L
Activity	Teaching centered and subject based	Student centered and problem based
Retention	In listening 10-20%	In doing 60-70%
Role	Teacher's ability to deliver goods is important	Student is an active learner, teacher is a facilitator
Number of students	Large group	Small group (6-8)
Monitoring	Individual student cannot be monitored	Can monitor individually
Type of learning	Passive learning	Active learning

OBJECTIVE OF PBT-L

In the current pharmacy professional scenario, the students should possess enhanced communication skills, greater problem-solving capabilities, effective critical thinking abilities and sound decision making skills. Pharmacy educators carry the responsibility of building above mentioned skills in the students through appropriate teaching-learning methodologies. This potential necessity led to the development of PBT-L approach in the pharmacy education. Consequently, the objective of PBT-L method is to build knowledge, skills and abilities in students that are required for them to be competent in the future pharmacy profession.

BENEFITS OF PBT-L

1) Reinforces the development of an effective process including the skills of problem synthesis, hypothesis generation and critical appraisal of available information, data analysis and decision making.
2) Develops an ability to identify relevant problems that demand further discussion or self-study within the context of a particular subject.

3) Cultivate the skills necessary to become self-directed learner with making effective use of available learning resources.
4) Helps to function effectively as an active participant within a small group engaged in learning.
5) Facilitate to recognize, develop and maintain the personal characteristics and attitudes necessary for a career in the pharmacy profession. These include the awareness of personal assets, limitations and emotional reactions, responsibility, dependability, the evaluation of personal progress and group process.
6) Develops creative and critical thinking, communication and collaborative working skills.

PROCESS OF PBT-L

In PBT-L method, the students are divided into small groups (each group containing 6-8 students) and a facilitator is expected to monitor and guide all the group's activities. The PBT-L process involves five key steps (design the problem, understand the problem, search strategies, resolve the problem, and evaluate the learning process). Each of these five key steps is completed by performing numerous sub-steps. The flow of PBT-L process is outlined in Figure 5.1.

A) Designing the problem: The designed problems should be curriculum based, able to provide active learning environment, and able to allow the students to gain broader knowledge. In addition, the designed problems should be such that subsequent learning should help in future work scenario. Generally, two kinds of problems (real or made problem) can be designed. The problem should be relevant to the curriculum and help to achieve the common goal of PBT-L. The designed problem should have the following features.

- Problem structure should inherently link to critical thinking. In other words, the problems should be ill-structured with just presenting the initial situation and stimulating the learners to generate multiple hypotheses about the cause and possible solution. This helps learners to achieve optimum development of critical thinking skills.

- Each problem should contain a "facilitator guide" that identifies a range of topics needing to address during the learning sessions. This guide should be kept with the facilitator and not given to students. At the end of a session, the facilitator is required to review the list of topics with the each member of the group.

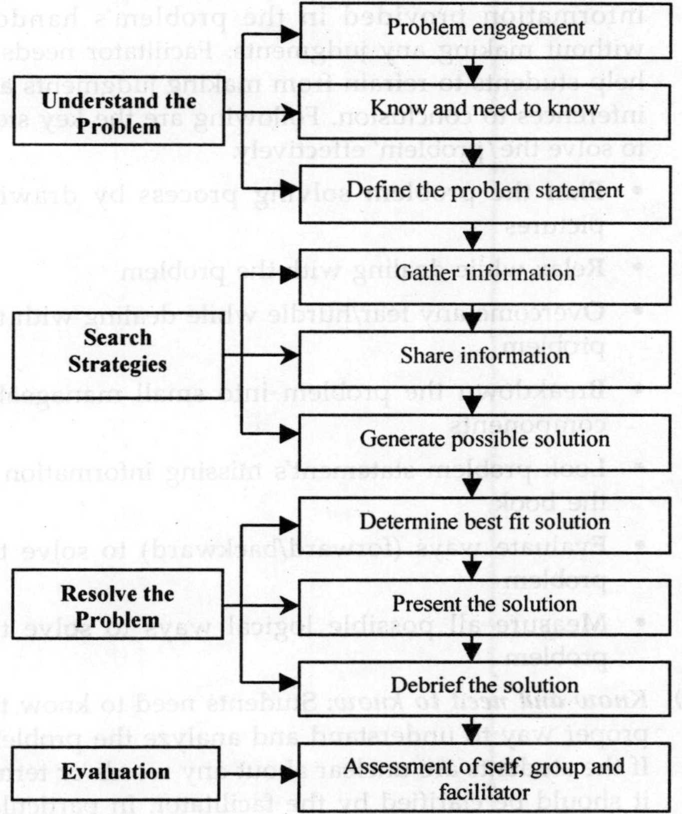

Figure 5.1. The schematic representation of PBT-L process

- The problem should ideally provoke inquiry and discussion on the concepts of related subjects (chemistry, pharmaceutics, anatomy, physiology, pharmacology, therapeutics and pathophysiology) of the curriculum.

B) Understand the problem

1) ***Engagement of the problem*:** Once the problem is designed, handouts of the problem need to be distributed to each member of the group. Then, students should list the objectives and key information provided in the problem's handout without making any judgments. Facilitator needs to help students to refrain from making judgments and inferences to conclusion. Following are the key steps to solve the 'problem' effectively.

   - Plan the problem solving process by drawing pictures
   - Relax while dealing with the problem
   - Overcome any fear/hurdle while dealing with the problem
   - Breakdown the problem into small manageable components
   - Look problem statement's missing information in the book
   - Evaluate ways (forward/backward) to solve the problem
   - Measure all possible logical ways to solve the problem

2) ***Know and need to know*:** Students need to know the proper way to understand and analyze the problem. If the students are unclear about any words or terms, it should be clarified by the facilitator. In particular, they need to understand the mechanisms that might

explain concepts associated with the problem. Students then need to assess the current understanding of the basic structural and/or functional mechanisms that may contribute to the presentation of the problem. After completing their own understanding, know/gather the collective skills and experiences of other members of the group to explore or explain the alternative phenomena.

3) ***Define the problem statement***: Facilitator should guide the students to frame the problem and generate hypotheses or statements of the possible causes for the issues presented in the problem. Students should first list the generated possibilities. Then, the group should prioritize the hypotheses from most likely to least likely hypotheses, followed by student's brainstorming on the subjective issues which in turn based upon the facts and their evolving knowledge. After generating hypotheses (learning issues), students are then need to determine if the additional information is required to solve the problem. At this stage, facilitator can present learning issues in the form of questions which helps students to generate the learning issues (hypotheses).

C) Search strategies

1) ***Gather information***: Once the learning issues are prioritized, the students need to identify the resources and then gather the information. Numerous resources can be used to gather the information (for example, books, previous class notes, research and review articles, discussion with experts, online resources, and databases). If it is clinical or patient based problem, then the possible resources are communication with the patient and family members, discussion with other health care professionals, patient records and observations (if the patient is available during the session).

2) *Share information*: Every student needs to share problem related knowledge, information, and personal opinions with other members of the group. At this stage, it is important for everyone in the group to communicate each other effectively. Student's communication skills can be improved through their active participation in the learning activity.

3) *Generate possible solution*: The group has to discuss how the researched information changes the view of the case. The most likely hypothesis is addressed in light of the new information and then students determine the necessity of additional information to understand and solve the problem. The hypotheses need to be narrowed down to a short list of probable solutions.

D) Resolve the problem

1) *Determine best fit solution*: After preparing a short list of probable solutions, the group has to select the most likely solution and discuss the rationale for the choice. Following are the key steps that help to determine the best solution and 'solve' the problem.

   - Select the most apparent logical solution
   - Organize your thought to reach an optimal solution
   - Locate other possible solutions to the problem, if any
   - Validate and verify the reached solution
   - Examine all possible solutions and choose the optimal one

2) *Present the solution*: In this stage, students need to share their understandings/views with other members of the group. It is helpful to begin with a brief survey of what each of them did to address the learning objectives identified by the group in the

previous session. Upon presentations, facilitator should encourage the students to refine their presentation and recommend for more precise presentations. In addition, the questions a facilitator might ask are: *a*) how might you quickly summarize what you have been saying?, *b*) what is a more precising way of saying that? and *c*) how could you better organize that to get your point across more effectively?

3) ***Debrief the solution*:** To finalize a solution with acceptable conclusion for the proposed problem, students are required to present their solutions and listen to other member's presentation. Then, all the information is brought together in the debriefing session, where students examine how the various solutions differed and why. In this stage, the students learn about different approaches to the problem by comparing their approaches with other's approaches. In addition, students also learn about general strategies for handling the problem.

E) **Evaluation—Self, group, problem and facilitator:** Each PBT-L session should end with the discussion about the progress of the session and fulfillment of set objectives. It is essential that the impact of this learning method be properly appraised. This is done by assessing the student's and facilitator's performances. All the participants are required to involve actively in the process of regular review of the PBT-L program. Alternatively, after completion of each session, facilitator needs to have an informal feed-back session (~ 10 minutes) to give feedback (positive or negative) on the effectiveness of the session (individually or group). The feedback provides both the students and facilitators an opportunity to know about the growth and development in their respective tasks. The group members should be encouraged to involve actively in the evaluation process and take the responsibility for initiating the change.

The assessment of student's and facilitator's performance in the PBT-L activity is done using all the modes given below.

1) ***Self assessment of student's participation***: The unique skills of PBT-L are preparation, responsibilities, participation, group skills, communication, professionalism, reflectiveness, critical thinking and teaching. Using the student's participation evaluation form (see Table 5.2), each student needs to perform the self-assessment of performance with respect to PBT-L skills using a scale of 1-5. Importantly, students should perform the self-assessment before the student's participation evaluation by a facilitator (see below).

2) ***Assessment of student's participation by a facilitator:*** Using the same student's participation evaluation form (see Table 5.2), facilitator needs to assess the performance of each student with respect to PBT-L skills using a scale of 1-5.

3) ***Assessment of facilitator's role by the students***: The students of each group needs to assess the facilitator's role by using a facilitator's role (behavior/character) evaluation form (see Table 5.3). In this assessment, students needs to state whether the facilitator's roles were helpful or not.

4) ***Assessment of facilitator's role by governing body***: In academia, there is an obligation to ensure that our peers uphold the standards of the profession. Therefore, the governing body needs to collect the facilitator's role assessment forms completed by the students, evaluate whether facilitators met the teaching standards or not, and give the feed-back to the facilitators. The facilitator's skills needing to improve should be informed and facilitate for self-development through practice.

Table 5.2

Student's participation evaluation form[a]

Please rate each member of your tutorial group by circling your choice on the following characteristics. Please give a copy to the student. Note: 1 is highest rating and 5 is lowest rating

Student:__________________; **Facilitator:**____________________ **Date:**__________

High to exceptional		Unsatisfactory to low
Consistently well-prepared for sessions: E.g., uses a variety of references; supports statements with appropriate references; makes concise summaries.	**PREPARATION** **1 2 3 4 5**	**Consistently seems unprepared for sessions:** E.g., inadequate reading or researching of learning issues: contributes little to group knowledge; does not summarize material.
Accepts responsibility for own learning: E.g., directs own learning agenda; actively tries to improve; critiques resources.	**RESPONSIBILITY** **12 3 4 5**	**Does not accept responsibility for own learning:** E.g., depends upon others for learning agenda; covers up mistakes; rarely critiques resources.
Active participation in group learning: E.g., actively participates in discussions; willingly takes on assignments.	**PARTICIPATION** **1 2 3 4 5**	**Passive participation in group learning:** E.g., does not actively participate in discussions: reluctantly takes on assignments.
Demonstrates effective group skills/awareness: E.g., takes the lead or intervenes appropriately; shows respect and sensitivity for others, helps to resolve misunderstandings and conflicts.	**GROUP SKILLS** **1 2 3 4 5**	**Demonstrates poor group skills/awareness:** E.g., intervenes inappropriately; shows poor judgment by interrupting, withdrawing, ignoring others, dominating or impatience.

Skillful in communicating with peers: E.g., listens actively; sensitive to non-verbal and emotional messages.	**COMMUNICATION** 1 2 3 4 5	**Difficulties communicating with peers:** E.g., poor listening skills; unable or unwilling to attend to non-verbal or emotional messages.
Highly developed professional behavior: E.g., excellent attendance; reliable; willingly accepts feedback and learns from it.	**PROFESSIONALISM** 1 2 3 4 5	**Deficiencies in professional behavior:** E.g., absent without an excuse; untrustworthy; difficulty in accepting feedback.
High self-awareness: E.g., recognizes limits of knowledge or abilities without becoming defensive or blaming others.	**REFLECTIVENESS** 1 2 3 4 5	**Low self-awareness:** E.g.. needs to be more aware of limitations in knowledge and ability and take positive steps toward remediation.
Highly skilled in critical thinking: E.g., consistently demonstrates skill in performing key tasks such as generating hypotheses, applying knowledge of PBT-L cases, critically appraising information, making sound deductions, explaining reasoning process.	**CRITICAL THINKING** 1 2 3 4 5	**Deficient in critical thinking:** E.g., consistent difficulties in performing key tasks such as generating hypotheses, applying knowledge of PBT-L cases, critically appraising information, making sound deductions, explaining reasoning process.
Effective teaching skills: Presents learning issue report at appropriate level, related to the case and in an organized fashion. Uses handouts or summaries to help others remember the material	**TEACHING** 1 2 3 4 5	**Ineffective teaching skills:** Presents learning issue report at inappropriate level, fail to relate material to the case and presents in a disorganized fashion. Fails to use handouts or summaries to help others remember the material

- Please add any comments (for example, strengths and weaknesses) about the person you are evaluating. Use the other side if necessary. [a] Based on Blake et al., Colliver, and Norman and Schmidt .

RESPONSIBILITIES OF STUDENTS AND FACILITATOR

In order to complete PBT-L session successfully, students and facilitator should know and fulfill their responsibilities efficiently. Following are the responsibilities of the students and facilitator.

Responsibilities of Students

- **Self-learning:** Self-learning is a highly essential skill for students which make them competitive in the pharmacy profession. Since the PBT-L is a student centred learning process, it is the responsibility of each student to participate actively and fully, not only for his or her learning, but also for supporting the learning of other members of the group. Although much of the student's time may be spent alone in the library or at the computer, the full benefits of PBT-L should not be realized in isolation. In this way, students can design their learning to meet their own needs (as everyone differs in knowledge and experience) and career aspirations. Facilitator needs to guide the students in assuming this key responsibility and prepare them to become effective and efficient life-long learners.
- **Integration of various disciplines:** Problem-based learning should not occur within a single discipline or subject. Instead, during self-directed learning, students should be able to access, study and integrate the information gathered from all the disciplines that might be useful in understanding and resolving the problem. This allows the students to learn better, recall and apply prior information of various relevant fields in their future work life.

Table 5.3

Facilitator's role evaluation form[a]

Facilitator: ______________________________ **Date:** ______________

Instructions to student: Behaviors or characteristics of facilitator are given below

- CIRCLE "1" if the facilitator's behavior was helpful to your (student's) learning or group process.
- CIRCLE "2" if it was unhelpful.
- CIRCLE "NA" if the occasion didn't arise for demonstration of this behavior.

Sl. No.	Behaviors/Characters	Helpful	Not Helpful	No Applicable
1	Encouraged thinking, inquiry and critical reasoning	1	2	NA
2	Encouraged a safe environment to express ignorance/ideas without fear of embarrassment	1	2	NA
3	Demonstrated sensitivity and respect for students.	1	2	NA
4	Struck a balance between providing information and actively involving students	1	2	NA
5	Provided feedback when appropriate	1	2	NA
6	Facilitated participation of all members of the group	1	2	NA
7	Refocused the group when discussion was wandering	1	2	NA
8	Encouraged and valued contributions from students	1	2	NA
9	Encouraged student responsibility for the learning objectives	1	2	NA
10	Questioned and probed the reasoning process	1	2	NA
11	Encouraged critical appraisal of information	1	2	NA
12	Encouraged students to assume leadership responsibilities	1	2	NA

For questions 13-15 use the following scale:

Sl.No.	Overall	Very high to Very low
13	Overall effectiveness of the tutor	1 2 3 4 5
14	Overall value to the facilitator	1 2 3 4 5
	Motivation	1 2 3 4 5
15	Motivation for problem-based learning is	1 2 3 4 5

16. **Open-ended comments:** Please describe any strengths or weaknesses of the PBT-L. Include any ideas about how the facilitator might improve.

[a] Based on Blake et al., Colliver, and Norman and Schmidt.

- **Creative thinking, collaboration and communication skills:** Students should be able to think critically on the problem and generated solutions to the problem. Critical thinking helps students to find a relevant information and solution independently. Further, while discussing about the gathered information and possible solutions to the problem, students should be able to collaborate and communicate effectively with other members of the group. Effective collaboration and communication build the self-confidence and self-learning ability in the students.

Responsibilities of Facilitator

PBT-L is task-oriented teaching-learning method. The objective of PBT-L is to build knowledge, skills and abilities in students that are required for being competent in the future pharmacy profession. Therefore, the facilitator should lead each group successfully to achieve the common goals of the PBT-L. To accomplish the common goals, facilitator needs to fulfill the following sub-responsibilities while conducting PBT-L sessions.

1) Select an appropriate problem by creating facilitator guide and specific objectives for each stage of the curriculum.

2) Should have abilities and skills relevant to the principles and practice of problem-based teaching-learning.

3) Assist the group to set early goals and tutorial plan which may be modified later including an organizational frame work and evaluation plan.

4) Guide the students to identify the key issues in the problem and find the ways to learn those areas in detail. The role of the facilitator in PBT-L is very different from the conventional teacher's role, in which teacher acts as a "content expert" who provides the facts.

5) Must be active and directive about the learning process to assure that the group achieves target and learn the key issues, without being a passive observer.

6) If the facilitator is an expert in an area where students are having trouble, act as a resource person to the group. However, leave the responsibility in the hands of the students. Don't guess if students are stuck and ask for your help, give them some assistance. This will certainly remove some frustration and helps students think about other important learning objectives.

7) It is essential for facilitator to be honest with students as students think facilitator as their role model.

8) Facilitator should encourage and motivate the slow learners to cope up with other participants.

9) The facilitator should fulfill responsibilities in the facilitator's role by attending the orientation/training workshops and meetings.

10) Help students to improve study methods including the collection of appropriate learning resources.

11) Review learning achievement and ensure that the student receive the timely feedback. This can be done by preparing the evaluation report on the individual student learning progress, including comments as to whether the student has or has not completed the objectives of the PBT-L.

12) Ask appropriate questions to facilitate learning. Questioning will keep the group focused and help students to present information and concepts more precisely. Facilitator should know how and when to ask appropriate questions. Following are some examples of questioning.
    - Ask open-ended questions to promote discussion rather than focusing on yes/no type questions or using quiz type questions.
    - Encourage students to make connection between two issues. For example, what is the association between hypertension and diabetes mellitus?
    - Periodically, ask students to define and explain the terminologies used in the problem. For example, what is sterilization? What are the different methods of sterilization?
    - Ask higher order questions. For example, what is the best treatment for this patient to treat diabetes mellitus? Why do we treat this condition? What is the mechanism of action of this drug? What is the evidence to justify significance of the treatment? How do you select the suitable laboratory tests?
13) Assess student's understanding and knowledge at different stages of PBT-L. This can be done by asking to draw a diagram to illustrate a concept, show the relationships among concepts, and summarize the discussion at particular stage of the session.

INNOVATIONS IN PBT-L

ICTs have been used as supportive tools or to replace the facilitator, thereby providing more flexible and improvised learning environment. Use of e-mail-based communication mode and computerization of PBT-L process are the innovations that have been adopted so far. The modifications in each of the revolutionized PBT-L methods (computerized PBT-L (CPBT-L) and e-mail assisted PBT-L methods) are discussed in detail below.

1) **Computerized PBT-L (CPBT-L):** In this revolutionized PBT-L method, computer is used to replace the facilitator-led group sessions (computerized PBT-L (CPBT-L)) or supplement traditional facilitator-led group sessions (computer supplemented PBT-L). In the traditional PBT-L sessions, the primary role of a facilitator is to guide, pose questions and provide appropriate corrective feedback and support to students. In the CPBT-L, facilitator's job has been simulated by a computer program and function as an "expert" tutor or facilitator. Substitution of facilitator-led group sessions by computerization substantially reduces personnel requirements for colleges with large class sizes. On the other hand, in computer supplemented PBT-L, students can use the computers to review PBT-L material at their own pace and provide (put-in) the responses. Computers can be used to incorporate video or multimedia experiences that would be difficult to demonstrate in person within individual groups. Facilitator expertise is advantageous for enhancing student learning in PBT-L sessions, particularly when a problem lacks sufficient structure or when the students lack prior knowledge of a subject. Thus, the computer can serve as a consistent source of expertise with respect to PBT-L case content. Following are ways to conduct the computerized PBT-L sessions.

***Design and development of computerized PBT-L case*:** Suitable software (for example, Authorware Professional™) has been used for case (problem) development. The computerized case is structured in a manner that allows students to complete all the steps in the PBT-L process normally performed in the facilitator-led group sessions (see process of PBT-L section). Two versions of the CPBT-L cases can be developed: *1*) CPBT-L cases without concept map material, and 2) CPBT-L cases with the addition of concept map material. Concept maps are schematic drawings in which individual concepts are connected by linking phrases and labeled to represent the relationships among them. The concept map promotes student's active and meaningful learning and motivation. Then, students need to review the problem scenario and let the computer to ask open-ended questions to clarify the situation. The computer is programmed to "match" keywords or phrases in the questions and either provide additional data in response, assist the students in resolving the questions themselves by guiding them through a series of prompts for which responses were needed (similar to what a facilitator might do during a group discussion), or refer them to references to find the needed information. All "unmatched" questions the students ask are automatically recorded by the computer to allow for future incorporation of new keywords. Students are then need to rank the hypotheses for the cause(s) of the problem, receive feedback and obtain helpful hints as needed to arrive at a reasonable option(s). As a part of the PBT-L process, students need to state a learning objective for the situation, type in potential ideas to resolve the problem, and prepare a plan of action.

Similar to facilitator-led PBT-L, CPBT-L also consists of written assignments at different stages of learning. The designed computer program is such that students may not be able to proceed into the hypotheses portion of the problem without a password. At this point, individual student will have to write down their hypotheses, rank order them, and turn them in. In addition, at selected level, the student's choices or responses is recorded. These data are also used as a measure of the student's problem-solving abilities, in lieu of direct facilitator observations of the groups.

2) **E-mail assisted problem based teaching-learning:** The traditional PBT-L requires the facilitator to be present for all group's meeting sessions. Increased facilitators requirement led to cost increment. As a result, although PBT-L is a powerful teaching-learning method, its implementation in the pharmacy education is often slowed by economic issue. Therefore, educators were searching for an alternative approach in which a facilitator can guide as many groups as possible. To overcome the economic issue, e-mail assisted PBT-L has been established. It is a simple and cost-effective approach to the traditional PBT-L which provides an efficient and economical means of communication between a facilitator and a large number of student discussion groups. A single teacher can serve as facilitator for 12-14 groups in the time it would normally take to work with two groups. This advanced (electronic) communication mode obviously reduced the personnel costs significantly associated with traditional PBT-L. The e-mail approach is feasible for conventional as well as some distance learning environments.

   In this approach, the class is taught with PBT-L activities implemented as out-of-class group projects. Briefly, facilitator needs to appoint a team representative who should then arrange the group meeting sessions and communicate questions or requests back to the facilitator through the class e-mail accounts. Once the problem is distributed as handouts or via e-mail, groups needs to meet in a convenient place to discuss about the problem, hypotheses, and possible solutions. Any unsolved questions can be asked to the facilitator via class e-mail account. The facilitator then needs to interact with the students by email. For expected student's queries, facilitator can interact with them by e-mail using a library of responses or modified responses. On the other hand, unexpected student's questions need to be answered individually. Ideally, for each problem, a group can meet 3-4 times and interact 3-4 times with the facilitator. However, these may vary depending on the problem scenario. All the responses need to be added to the response library. E-mail assisted PBT-L makes very efficient use of the facilitator's time without compromising the fundamental advantages of PBT-L.

REFERENCES

1. Cutler TW, Stebbins MR, Lai E, Smith AR, Lipton HL. 2008. Problem-based learning using the online medicare Part D plan finder tool. American Journal of Pharmaceutical Education 72:1-8.
2. Brueggemeier RW. 1998. Perspectives on the future of graduate education in medicinal chemistry and pharmacognosy. American Journal of Pharmaceutical Education 62:463-467.
3. Haworth IS, Eriksen SP, Chmait SH, Matsuda LS, McMillan PA, King EA, Wagner JL, Shapiro K. 1998. A problem based learning, case study approach to pharmaceutics: Faculty and student perspectives. American Journal of Pharmaceutical Education 62:398-405.
4. Herrier RN, Jackson TR, Consroe PF. 1997. The use of Student centred, problem based, clinical case discussion to enhance learning in pharmacology and medicinal chemistry. American Journal of Pharmaceutical Education 61:441-446.
5. Wilms LR. 2001. Innovative enabling strategies in self-directed, problem-based therapeutics: Enhancing student preparedness foe pharmaceutical care practice. American Journal of Pharmaceutical Education 65:56-64.
6. Fisher RC. 1994. The potential for problem-based learning in pharmacy education: A clinical therapeutics course in Diabetes. American Journal of Pharmaceutical Education 58:183-189.

7. Blake RL, Hosokawa MC, Riley SL. 2000. Student performances on Step 1 and Step 2 of the United States medical licensing examination following implementation of a problem-based learning curriculum. Academic Medicine 75:66-70.

8. Colliver JA. 2000. Effectiveness of problem-based learning curricula: Research and theory. Academic Medicine 75:259-266.

9. Norman GR, Schmidt HG. 2000. Effectiveness of problem-based learning curricula: Theory, practice and paper darts. Medical Education 34:721-728.

10. Maudsley G. 1999. Roles and responsibilities of the problem based learning tutor in the undergraduate medical curriculum. British Medical Journal 318: 657-661.

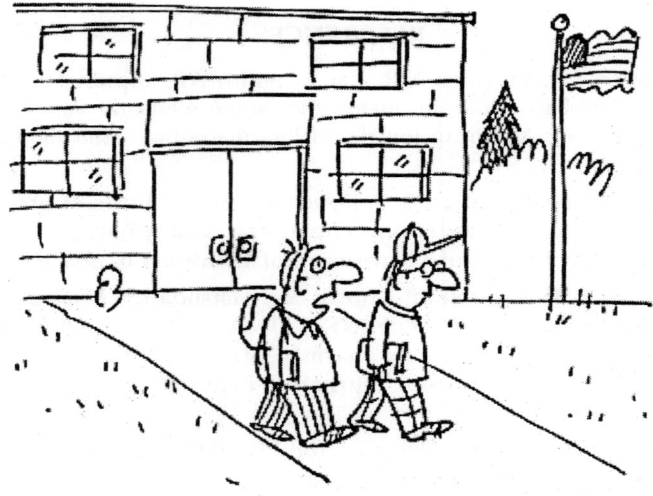

"I don't get it! They make us learn reading, thinking, writing, and discussing to prepare us for a world of technologies"

Chapter 6

CASE BASED TEACHING-LEARNING

Shobha Churi

"The greatest pleasure in life is doing what people say you cannot do"

—Walter Bagehot

Case based teaching-learning (CBT-L) is an educational format utilizing 'real life' case/problem/inquiry to create an active and collaborative learning environment. Writing, delivering and examining/analyzing a case, brainstorming, formulating learning objectives, dissemination of new findings, sharing the results by the group, and identifying the areas for improvement and integrating into the next process are the stages of CBT-L program. CBT-L method provides an opportunity to students to develop self-learning, creative and critical thinking, collaborative and self-evaluative skills.

INTRODUCTION

As pharmacy profession is becoming more and more advanced and highly competitive, greater competencies (self-learning, creative thinking, collaborative, critical thinking, self-evaluative skills etc.) skills are expected from pharmacy graduates. Further, pharmacy subject's problem solving has been considered as a complex phenomenon. Educators are now adopting potential educational methods to solve the complex problems and build the essential competencies in students. The basic objective of using novel methods is to build/strengthen the knowledge upon which the students can overcome the future problems in their professional career. Among the methods adopted, problem based teaching-learning (PBT-L) and CBT-L methods have been most effective in fulfilling the above mentioned objective.

CBT-L is an educational format which is closely related to the more common PBT-L method. Although both the methods (PBT-L and CBT-L methods) are closely related, CBT-L approach comprises of distinct characteristics as shown in Table 6.1. CBT-L is an educational format utilizing 'real life' case/problem/inquiry of the pharmacy subjects to create an active and collaborative learning environment. Cases place events in a context or situation that promote authentic learning. Cases are generally written or designed as problems that provide the student with a background of a topic/situation. Supporting information is provided, such as latest research articles and other related information/results. CBT-L approach creates the situation in which students collects the information, apply theory or technique, or follow particular analytical or decision making procedures. Due to enormous success gained over few decades, CBT-L approach is being used to teach a variety of pharmacy subjects. The reasons for success are the benefits that are being offered by the CBT-L method (see below).

BENEFITS/ADVANTAGES OF CBT-L METHOD

1) Allows students to develop a collaborative, team based approach to their education.
2) Students generate hypothesis, consolidate and integrate into the learning activities, thereby acquiring these skills.
3) Students develop intrinsic and extrinsic motivation skills, thereby become self-learners.
4) Encourages self-evaluation and critical reflection.

5) Allows students for scientific inquiry and the development of support provision for their conclusions.
6) Integrates knowledge and practice.
7) Develops learning skills.
8) Enhances student's confidence.

Table 6.1
A comparison between PBT-L and CBT-L methods

PBT-L	CBT-L
Initial topic	
• Unknown to students.	• General content is disclosed to students.
Preparation	
• Students do not prepare themselves in advance for the learning process.	• Students prepare themselves in advance for the learning process.
Control	
• Students do not provide any direction. Directly involve in discussion.	• Students provide some direction.
• Teacher provides no direction to control the process.	• Teacher provides some direction to control the process.
Data seeking	
• Students seek lots of additional data during or after problem.	• Students seek some additional data during or after case.
• Teacher seeks some additional data during or after problem.	• Teacher does not seek additional data during or after case.

CHALLENGES OF CBT-L METHOD

Along with numerous benefits, CBT-L method presents few challenges that must be overcome by the educators. Educators need to adopt modified or alternative or novel strategies to overcome the following challenges.

1) CBT-L approach can be more demanding in terms of staff time and workload than traditional methods.

2) It might also be more demanding of resources (e.g. case study packs).
3) Students may be unprepared for the more active role demanded of them and may therefore not be able to gain the potential benefits.
4) Tutors may feel that their traditional role as 'expert' is challenged or undermined and will need to recognize 'a loss of power and control'.
5) Assessing CBT-L work can present new challenges and opportunities.

CBT-L PROCESS

The schematic representation of CBT-L process is shown in Figure 6.1. The key aspects of CBT-L process are discussed below.

1) **Writing a case:** A good case can be written by completing four key steps as given below.

a) ***Selection and design of story/problem*:** Following are essential characteristics of a case.

1) The case content should be closely aligned with the overall instructional goals and objectives.
2) The case should tell a story and focus on an issue that stimulates interest.
3) The case should be well-written and its readability should be appropriate for the age or level of the student.
4) The case should be written in the present tense and able to deal with an authentic situation not more than five years old.
5) The case should include direct quotes using the character's dialog to tell the story.
6) The story should be compelling and able to create empathy with the main characters.

7) The case should clearly state and illuminate the dilemma without resolving it.

8) The case should be relevant to the reader.

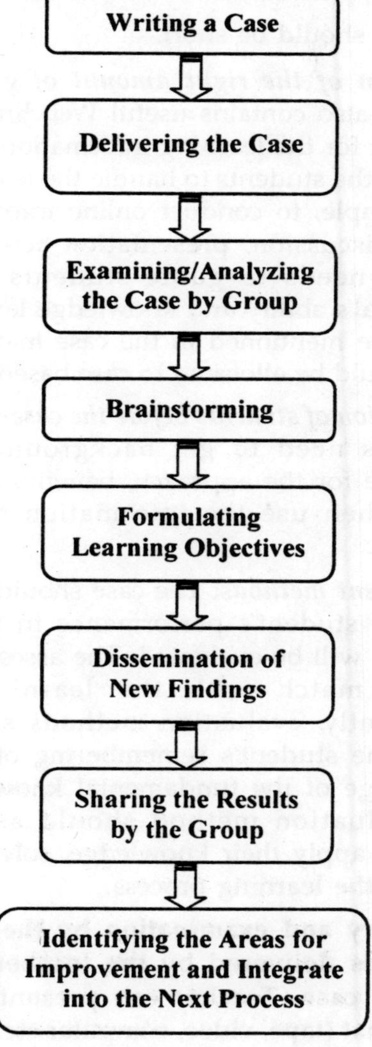

Figure 6.1. CBT-L Process (based on Williams B (2004))

9) The case should provoke conflict and force decision making.

10) The case should be general enough to be used in several applications.

11) The case should be short.

b) ***Provision of the right amount of guidelines***: Case material also contains useful Web links for students to search for the learning information. Teachers need to guide the students to handle the learning activities. For example, to conduct online information search, group discussion, presentation activities. Further, teacher needs to guide students based on the individual's ability and knowledge level. Time frame should be mentioned in the case material and more time should be allocated to case based activities.

c) ***Preparation of students before the case-based activities***: Teachers need to get background information (rationale for the approach, benefits etc) about CBT-L and then use the information to prepare the students.

d) ***Assessment methods***: The case should finally contain how the student's performance in the case based activities will be evaluated. The assessment methods should match with the learning objectives. Importantly, evaluation methods should not just assess the student's remembering of facts or basic knowledge of the fundamental knowledge. Instead, the evaluation method should assess how the students apply their knowledge, solve the case, and manage the learning process.

2) **Case delivery and examination by the group:** In this stage, case is delivered by the teacher and students analyze the case. Teacher can present the case in a suitable format (tape, video, computer etc.). Then, teacher and students need to perform certain roles to conduct case based learning process.

a) ***Roles of teacher***: Teacher plays multiple roles in the case based teaching. For example, he/she can be student, listener, questioner and analyst. Generally, teacher roles come under two broad general categories: *1*) setting up the learning environment (arranging chairs in a proper set-up (circle or horseshoe or some other configuration) that is favorable to discussion, establishing a friendly environment for open discussion, making clear the ground rules for open and respectful debate and good teacher's behavior) and *2*) facilitating discussion and exploration. Facilitating student discussion may appear to be simple, but in reality requires the teacher to use great skills in helping students explore and discuss the case in ways that maximize their learning. Following are some tips for facilitating the discussion effectively.

- Ask questions that encourage better thinking. At the same time, reveal the relevance of the discussion that has gone on before.
- Weave together the threads of individual contributions into a pattern the class can perceive.
- Use a good sense of timing for holding the discussion. Discussion should not be too fast for all students to comprehend.
- Exercise control over an essentially "undirected" activity while staying out of the way.
- Teacher should fill in with relevant information and be able to direct students to resources appropriate to the topic.

b) ***Roles of students***

- *Preparation for the case based process*: Students should prepare by reading cases and describing the issues, perceptions and possible courses of action. The student should also review literature relevant to the case.

- *Evaluation of a case and solutions*: Student should continually evaluate the case and proposed solutions. Then, reflect on what is learned and what needs to be learned. By evaluating and reflecting, the student takes more control of his or her own learning.
- *Participation*: Student must commit to collaborative work with peers.

EVALUATION OF CBT-L PROGRAM

Assessment and performance evaluation in CBT-L may seem daunting. It can be more subjective than some other educational evaluation methods. However, with careful lesson planning and preparation, assessment in CBT-L can be done efficiently, effectively and fairly. Following are the methods that can be used to assess the student's performances in CBT-L program.

1) Peer evaluation (student to student).
2) Periodic evaluation of key course elements.
3) Periodic evaluation of student's performance by the teacher.

The modes of assessment include: *a*) oral examination/ presentation, *b*) written examination (quizzes, multiple choice questions etc), and *c*) survey based on the teacher's and student's point-of-view. The student's performance assessment methods should include the standards and evaluation criteria as listed in Table 6.2. In case of a survey method, a questionnaire with questions pertaining to the CBT-L criteria should be prepared. Then, either student-to-student or teacher-to-student assessment is performed. The students or teachers are required to indicate the extent to which they agree or disagree with each of the questions using a five-point Likert-type scale ranging from strongly disagree to strongly agree (1 = strongly disagree, 2 = disagree, 3 = neutral, 4 = agree, and 5 = strongly agree). Finally required statistical data can be calculated.

TYPES OF CBT-L

CBT-L can occur in variety of ways as given below.

1) Written CBT-L in a classroom: Written cases can range from a short sketch used to illustrate a theoretical point to elaborate cases, presented in sections, with questions to help students develop practical thinking patterns and integrate theoretical content. The cases typically include a brief overview or descriptive information that both establishes a context for the problem and identify major decisions that must be made. The cases need to integrate concepts covered in the teaching portion of the course. These kinds of cases help students to achieve high-level learning involving analysis and synthesis of knowledge.

For CBT-L, cases are provided to student's groups (each group comprising 4-6 students). Each student should be assigned with a defined role. Each assignment needs to be completed between 1-2 weeks. In the first meeting on each assignment, students need to review the case, identify associated learning issues, discuss the accompanying questions, brainstorm possible solutions, delineate appropriate resources, and divide the responsibilities among the group members. The teacher needs to facilitate this process by providing ready access to relevant resource materials on-site. This task can be accomplished by providing resource materials including books, journal articles and other relevant informational resources on a mobile cart. Most information is usually derived from the recommended references, multiple copies of which are placed on the cart. Students are required to share information freely with group members. This allows students to acquire new information and resolve potential conflicts and dilemmas. During the each assignment, the group leader needs to interact with the teacher. All the groups can pursue the cases outside of the classroom by meeting at mutually convenient times as needed. Once the students acquire additional information, they can meet again to share

Table 6.2: Standards and criteria for student's performance assessment in CBT-L program[a]

Impact	Standard	Criteria
Student Behavior	Intellectual Development	Quality of thinking
	Skills	Communication, research and interpersonal skills.
	Attitudes	Personal perspectives, beliefs and values, self-evaluation.
Generative Activities	Projects	Evidence of research; analysis of information; organization & layout; creativity and originality.
	Written and Oral Presentations	Organization; fresh perspective; use of examples; development of ideas; use of facts to substantiate arguments; quality of thought and analysis.
	Field Study	Hypothesis; systematic data collection; relevance of conclusions; identification of relationships.
	Making Comparisons	Ability to zero in on significant factors; extensive comparison.
	Applying Principles	Recognize principles or rules that apply; logical connection of principles and situations.

Analytical Activities	Evaluating and Judging	Specific, reasonable, sound and appropriate criteria; clear relationship.
	Interpreting	Comprehension of big ideas; analyses focused on important meaning; articulation of importance; discernment of implicit content and making inferences; speculation presented with caution.
	Summarizing	Reflection of key ideas; succinct, accurate representation of key issues; articulate and intelligible summaries.
	Classifying	Connected attributes; larger purpose; enable new meaning; beyond the obvious.
	Decision-Making	Articulated values behind choices; humanly sound values; informed choice using best available data; carefully thought out.
	Creating and Inventing	Cognitive risks; truly new, fresh and imaginative; appropriate to demands of the task.
	Designing Investigations	Frame problem for thoughtful investigation; logical, thoughtful investigation plans; data will yield information about the problem; viability; built-in evaluation; clear relationship between plan and problem.

[a]Based on Wasserman (1994)

new information in an attempt to seek a reasonable solution to the problems at hand.

Example: Stability kinetics

Mr. 'X' is working as a clinical Pharmacist at 'Y'. Mr. 'X' received a prescription that requires 1 g of cefazolin sodium to be administered to the patient in 100 mL of 0.9 % w/v normal saline (NS). Cefazolin is an antibiotic, which may be administered by slow infusion into the vein (IV infusion). Cefazolin is a weak acid (MW = 455; pKa = 2.1) and is poorly soluble in aqueous IV infusion solutions such as 5 % w/v dextrose or NS. Recognizing the solubility problem with cefazolin, Mr. 'X' prepared the formulation using the sodium salt of cefazolin (molecular weight = 477). When Mr. 'X' referred American hospital formulary services drug information to check the stability of the two marketed formulations of cefazolin sodium, Ancef® and Kefzol®, he learned that these solutions are stable for 10 days when refrigerated. Suspecting the stability of sodium cefazolin in aqueous solution at room temperature, Mr. 'X' sent his formulation to 'Z' for stability assessment. When assayed approximately 75 hours after the formulation has been prepared, the concentration of cefazolin found to be 8.4 mg/mL. The drug has been reported to undergo first-order degradation with a half-life of 12 days.

Questions

1) What would be the pH when 1 g of sodium cefazolin is dissolved and made up to a liter with purified water?
2) Do you expect that the pH of an admixture prepared in 5 % w/v dextrose or NS would be any different than the above aqueous preparation?
3) What is the rate constant for the first-order reaction, K?

4) What is the concentration remaining after 24 and 72 days?
5) What should be the expiration date on the label?
6) What fraction of drug will be remaining after 5 half-lives?
7) If the drug undergoes zero-order degradation with the same rate constant, what will be the half-life?
8) Does the pH of the formulation change when the concentration is dropped to 8.4 mg/mL
9) What is "accelerated stability analysis?" Explain how it is done.

2) Web-based module: Using the Internet technology, appropriate Web-based case study module has been developed for teaching the various subjects (for example, disease-based education, pharmacokinetics study etc.). Web-based study module can be designed using software design elements such as hypertext mark-up language (HTML) language and standard browser viewing. The Web-based module is organized into different phases of learning (for example, entering the blood glucose level, diagnostic, treatment, follow-up etc.) to assure that a student clusters the actions needed for each particular phase. Various personnel (for example, students, teachers, doctors and patients) and systems are involved in each phase of the process, thereby illustrating collaboration. In addition, a student is challenged to define the outcomes and time frames for the next plan.

The design and navigation procedures of the module engage the students and ease them through the scenarios. The information in the modules is of two types: literature-based and case-based. The Web cases incorporate menu bars, electronic feedback, faculty and student group meetings and electronic mail among students. The menu bar provides access to the various data sources needed for reasoning and decision-making. Electronic feedback occurs in response to student choices. There can be virtual discussions among students through electronic mail and students can view peer responses in selected situations and provide feedback to one another.

3) **Patient case module:** This module is particularly useful in teaching the clinical and community pharmacy subjects. Teaching-learning occur with the real patients suffering from a disease/illness/disorder. Briefly, students study the patient's history and treatment given. Additionally, they needs to interact with the patients and doctors which can be videotaped. Then, students and faculty needs to view their videotape/student's presentation and discuss about the cause and possible solution. This module provides an opportunity for students to have face-to-face interactions with patients and deal with the real problem, thereby gaining experience with clinical reasoning.

4) **Computerized case module:** Computerized case study module has been developed using appropriate software (Microsoft Visual Basic 3.0 for example). Computerized case study module is a multifaceted decision tree. Since the design of computerized case study varies with topic/subject, case structure and format is explained here by taking an example (medicinal chemistry based case). In computerized case based teaching-learning method, students are presented with the initial case scenario and asked to answer an opening key question (e.g., which drug structure of the choices provided would be most appropriate to address a patient's therapeutic and personal needs?). After selecting the response to the initial key question, students are guided through the chemical thinking processes that allow them to arrive at the correct response. This task is accomplished by posing the questions that address desired or anticipated therapeutic outcomes and answer choices which give chemically-based explanations for these clinical responses. Students

are expected to analyze how specific chemical functional groups and/or physicochemical properties influence receptor affinity and selectivity, distribution, metabolic vulnerability, in vitro stability, potential route(s) of administration, and patient compliance. Drug structures, rather than drug names, are provided so that chemical reasoning motivates student response to case questions.

Wrong responses to case study questions commonly generate a series of new questions which guide students in discovering where their thinking went awry. Students who select wrong answers are often encouraged to consult appropriate volumes in the tutorial library before continuing with the case. To promote student acceptance of the program, the language utilized in the case study text and in the tutorials is conversational and, when appropriate, humorous. Positive reinforcement for correct responses is the rule. Computer-assisted teaching is the ideal format for the development of case studies which require integration of scientific and clinical reasoning. The advantages of computerized case study method are: *a*) it permits students to work at their own pace, and advance to more difficult cases when they are ready, *b*) supplementary information to assist students in solving case study problems can be loaded with the program, making a quick review of principles convenient, and *c*) it frees students from the anxiety of being wrong, since the mistakes they will inevitably make as problem-solving skills development can be corrected privately.

REFERENCES

1. Williams B. 2004. The implementation of problem-based learning and case-based learning: Shaping the pedagogy in ambulance education-A MUCAPS experience. In: Australian College of Ambulance Professionals. Alice Springs, Australia.
2. Wasserman S. 1994. Introduction to case method teaching: A guide to the galaxy. Teachers College Press, New York, USA.

3. Currie BC, Roche VF, Zito SW. 1996. Medicinal chemistry case study workbook. Williams and Wilkins, Baltimore, MD, USA.

4. Flynn A, Klein J. 2001. The influence of discussion groups in a case-based learning environment. Educational Technology Research and Development 49:71-86.

5. David DK. 1954. Forward In McNair MP (Ed.). The case method at the Harvard business school. McGraw-Hill (p.viii), New York,USA.

6. Yadav A, Lundeberg M, DeSchryver M, Dirkin K, Schiller N, Maier K, Herreid C. 2007. Teaching science with case studies: A national survey of faculty perceptions of the benefits and challenges of using cases. Journal of College Science Teaching 37: 34-38.

Chapter 7

ELECTRONIC (E)-TEACHING-LEARNING BASICS AND METHODS

Kashappa Goud H. Desai

"The new electronic interdependence recreates the world in the image of a global village"

—Marshall McLuhan

INTRODUCTION

Generally speaking, e-teaching-learning is an advanced technological educational format which utilizes all electronic media (audio/video tape, internet, intranets, extranets, compact disc read-only memory (CD-ROM), computer, satellite broadcast and interactive TV) for information/knowledge delivery, interaction or facilitation. The most advanced and potential e-teaching-learning methods are: *a*) computer assisted teaching-learning, *b*) Web based teaching-learning, *c*) online teaching-learning, *d*) mobile teaching-learning, and *e*) pharmacy informatics. E-teaching-learning may be synchronous or asynchronous or a combination.

UNIQUE FEATURES OF E-TEACHING-LEARNING METHODS

1) Student centered teaching-learning methods.
2) Provides an opportunity for students to regulate the learning pace (self-paced learning). As per the need, students can speed up or slow down the learning pace.

3) Successful, proven and tested educational methods.
4) Provides instant learning, evaluation and feedback for the further development.
5) Involves variety of delivery methods suitable for different students, thereby providing multiple learning styles. This is more effective for certain students.
6) Eliminates geographical barriers. Faculty from across the globe can be involved in teaching-learning.
7) Allows students to choose study content and tools appropriate to their differing interests, needs and skill levels, thereby facilitating the self-directed learning.
8) Fosters greater interaction and collaboration among the students.
9) Learning process is accessible at all times (24/7). This makes scheduling easy and allows a greater number of students to attend classes.
10) Since the access is on-demand, learning is more precise.
11) Reduces the student costs.
12) Reduces institutional/university cost significantly.
13) Fosters greater student-teacher contact. It enhances student's and teacher's computer and internet skills.
14) Gives highest course completion rate/lowest drop out rate.
15) Reduces learning time.

DISADVANTAGES TO THE INSTITUTION/UNIVERSITY

1) The investment cost required for establishing e-teaching-learning is larger due to development costs. Institution/university needs to find the ways to acquire funds.
2) Institution/university faces numerous technology issues including whether the existing technology

infrastructure can accomplish the training goals, whether additional technological expenditures can be justified, and whether compatibility of all software and hardware can be achieved.

3) Existence of inappropriate content for e-teaching-learning.

4) Cultural acceptance is an issue in institutions/ universities where student demographics and psychographics may incline them against using educational technologies at all and let alone for e-learning.

DISADVANTAGES TO THE STUDENTS

1) The most common technological issues of the students are technophobia and unavailability of required technologies.

2) In spite of numerous innovations (network linking points, notebook computers, personal digital assistant, and mobile phones), methods does not rival that of printed workbooks or reference material.

3) Reduces social and cultural interaction. The impersonality, suppression of communication mechanisms such as body language, and elimination of peer-to-peer learning that are part of this potential disadvantage are lessening with advances in communications technologies.

METHODS OF E-TEACHING-LEARNING

E-teaching-learning covers variety of advanced teaching-learning methods (see below).

1) Computer assisted teaching-learning
2) Web-based teaching-learning
3) Online teaching-learning (purely online - no face-to-face meetings)
4) Mobile teaching-learning

5) Pharmacy informatics
6) Blended teaching-learning (combination of online and face-to-face)
7) Synchronous learning
8) Asynchronous learning
9) Teacher-led group learning
10) Self-study
11) Self-study with subject matter expert
12) Learning with video/audio tape

However, in the forthcoming chapters, only the basics of e-teaching-learning (information and communication technologies (ICTs) in pharmacy education: need, vision, goals, and ways to achieve, teaching-learning with ICTs: integration and evaluation, and impact of ICTs on students, teachers and educational institutions) and important teaching-learning methods (computer assisted teaching-learning, Web-based teaching-learning, online teaching-learning, mobile teaching-learning, and pharmacy informatics) are discussed.

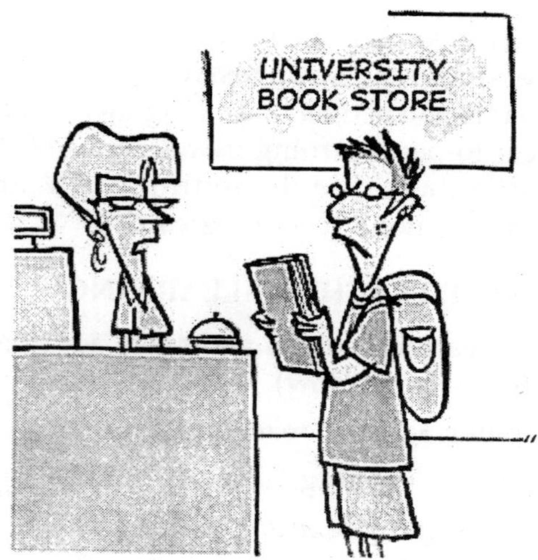

No, I don't have a scanner you can borrow."

Chapter 8

INFORMATION AND COMMUNICATION TECHNOLOGIES IN PHARMACY EDUCATION: NEED, VISION, GOALS AND WAYS TO ACHIEVE

Kashappa Goud H. Desai

"Technology means the systematic application of scientific or other organized knowledge to practical tasks"

—J. K. Galbraith

NEED FOR INNOVATIONS

Students of 21st century require the knowledge and skills that can enable them to be creative and enterprising. In addition, students need to be technologically competent, capable of using the opportunities of the digital world and self-managing of technology-based pharmacy careers that may change many times. Initiative, risk-taking, lateral thinking and resourcefulness are vital to the success. Rapid advancement in information and communication technologies (ICTs) is revolutionizing the pharmacy education worldwide. Portable electronic devices, network database applications, electronic pharmacy records and computer software programs have already been integrated into pharmacy educational system. The innovative and powerful technological tools, particularly ICTs, have been effective in creating a dynamic, student-centered and real-life problem based teaching-learning environment in educational institutions. With these advancements (ICTs-based teaching-learning), the pharmacy education is now moving to a new level. These changes are creating the need for other pharmacy institutions to become proficient using ICTs to deliver high-quality pharmacy education and services. Following are the key rationales for using ICTs in pharmacy education.

1) **Educational productivity:** There has been a growing need for the 'paradigm shift' in existing teaching methods to improve the quality of pharmacy education. Educational productivity is the ratio of the educational outcomes to the cost of teaching (see equation 1).

$$\text{Educational Productivity} = \frac{\text{Educational outcomes (quality and quantitiy of student learning)}}{\text{Costs (teacher and student time, classroom materials, equipment, etc.)}} \qquad (1)$$

It is apparent from the above equation that to increase the educational productivity, the outputs must increase and inputs must decrease. The innovative tools (ICTs) are necessary for improving the quality of student's learning. However, it is difficult to estimate the value of educational outcomes. Alternatively, the impact of ICTs on concepts of educational productivity can be considered. If the student's learning is improved through the use of appropriate ICTs, it suggests an increase in the value of the outcomes.

2) **ICTs solve problems:** The computers and communication technologies have become necessary to solve not only curriculum-embedded problems but also problems that occur during the regular curriculum. Therefore, the computers and communication technologies must be applied to pharmacy institution's problems such as those concerning teaching-learning (e.g., computer assisted learning, computerized problem based learning, teaching with multimedia, online lecture, teaching-learning with

other ICTs etc), administration (communication modes, leadership capacities) and so on. Following are the educational problems where ICTs play crucial role in overcoming the challenges.

- ***Student's learning***: ICTs are necessary to support student's learning activities which are difficult to perform in other ways. For example, to learn the complex topics of pharmacy disciplines (pharmacokinetics, pharmacology experiments, molecular drug design etc.), ICTs are highly necessary. These also act as stimulation and motivation tools for a range of learning activities.
- ***Management of learning experience***: Educators face numerous management problems while handling the educational data. Many of the teacher's tasks are time consuming and tedious. Hence, to maintain high-quality educational programmes, institution requires ICTs to handle the large quantities and types of data. Depending on the requirement, numerous ICTs packages can be developed and implemented. Educational institutions should make use of the technological tools to continually provide more appropriate solutions to the dynamic problems.
- ***Provision of support materials***: The access to, and production of, resource materials associated with the teaching-learning processes can be readily facilitated by the use of ICTs.
- ***Access information***: Students needs to respond to the mass of information and keep in touch with national and international experts for their ideas/opinions. It is an economical rationale to bring the efficient information to the students and teachers. Through the World Wide Web, new ideas and information can be accessed and transmitted instantly anywhere in the world with a click of a mouse. ICTs are required not only to provide speedy access to information but

also useful to process and interpret the information, to make meaning and present information.

3) **Other:** Changes to accreditation requirements may take place in the near future. The changes might ask pharmacy educational institutions to associate outcome measures with educational objectives of the program to enable assessment of student competencies.

INNOVATIVE VISION

"Expanding and improving the quality of pharmacy education with the help of ICTs and preparing the students for the future technological age."

INNOVATIVE GOALS AND WAYS TO ACHIEVE

1) **Empowering students with ICTs:** In this information age, students need to acquire the necessary skills, knowledge and attitudes for lifelong learning and creative problem solving. Students need to know the role of ICTs in various fields of study. For instance, computer assisted learning (computer-assisted pharmacology experiments for example), Web-based pharmacokinetics teaching, computerized distance learning for PharmD degree program, online lecture, Web-based clinical trials and use of information technology to avoid medication errors and improve the patient's safety. To learn the numerous topics, students need to understand the use of ICTs as information retrieval, knowledge inquiry, communication, collaboration, analytical and personal development tools. To empower the students with ICTs, the sub-goals such as framing the ICTs embedded curriculum, developing the assessment tools and providing the enhanced curriculum and learning materials (going beyond textbook) should be achieved.

   a) ***Curriculum—Clear learning objectives needed***

      • Pharmacy institutions/universities need to put significant effort in conceptualizing and embedding ICTs in the curriculum guides. For example, the role and relationship of ICTs in understanding the concepts of pharmacy subjects (for example, drug's pharmacokinetics, pharmacology experiments, drug design, clinical trials, pharmacy informatics, and avoiding the medication errors can be better understood/done with the use of ICTs). In addition, role of ICTs in providing an interactive learning environment also needs to be included.

- Institutions/universities and teachers should be guided on integration of ICTs into teaching-learning inside/outside classrooms with a view to cultivate the skills, knowledge and attitudes in students for lifelong learning. Students should be given with the opportunity to make use of ICTs to work collaboratively with peers as well as to identify and seek input and advice from people of different sectors in the community (local and international). For example, online lectures, Web-based learning, video conferencing and mobile learning. This can be achieved through the ways given below.

a) A broad framework of "ICTs literacy" for students should be developed to help teachers and students to have a clearer picture on the learning objectives of using ICTs in pharmacy education. The required ICTs literacy are: *1*) basic operations and concepts of ICTs, including when to use what tools and when not to use, *2*) social and ethical issues relating to the use of ICTs, *3*) use of ICTs as productivity, communication, collaboration, research and decision-making tools, *4*) strategies and skills for information retrieval and critical evaluation of different information sources, *5*) use of ICTs tools for information management and data analysis, and 6) knowledge management concepts and practices to support sustained work and collaboration.

b) Guidance should be developed on the application of ICTs in developing whole-institution/university curricula. This can be done by taking the successful cases of using ICTs in teaching-learning. In addition, such guidance should include both exemplary and suggested use of ICTs for teaching-learning in various subjects and be drawn up in consultation with teachers and experts.

c) For project-based and collaborative learning and other cross-curricular activities, interactive tool kits (e.g. using online learning platform) should be produced in institutions/universities. Teachers should be encouraged to share their prototypes with others and collaborate among themselves.

b) Assessment tools—Help teachers know student's learning outcome

- In order to assess student's attainment on the learning targets outlined under the ICTs framework, one should develop appropriate assessment tools to be used by teachers. The assessment should be performance-based and fully integrated with ICTs-enriched methodology that focuses on learner empowerment. The assessment should also provide teachers with formative evaluation information on the ICTs-enriched methodology employed.

- If universities/pharmacy institutions adopt the outcome-based approach for over a period of time, at least 25% of the curriculum to be taught with the support of ICTs may not be necessary. In this way, institutions should focus rightly back on students, not on the amount of teaching time with ICTs.

c) ***Curriculum and learning materials—Going beyond textbooks***

- As per the ICTs-embedded curriculum, universities/institutions should extend the spectrum of learning materials for their students to find resources to help them understand concepts, acquire knowledge and observe and explore the world outside university/institution. Further, universities/institutions should collaborate with other universities/ institutions worldwide to promote the use of ICTs in learning amongst students.
- The provision of suitably designed electronic (e)-learning platforms is necessary. Designed e-learning should support/enable students to engage in empowering modes of learning which include collaboration, inquiry and production of knowledge products. Management should support research and evaluation to identify appropriate educational e-learning platforms, provide teacher training, and enhance courseware in this regard.

2) **Empowering teachers with ICTs:** Universities/ institutions should provide a set of opportunities to teachers for professional development and support to undertake the challenge of using ICTs for curriculum and teaching innovations. In addition, universities/ institutions should support teachers to facilitate, guide, administer and assess learning in ways that align with the goals of the curriculum reform. Universities/ institutions should develop support structures and mechanisms to encourage the development of online and off-line communities of pharmacy for teachers for exchanging experience and collaborated problem solving activity. Following are the some ways to empower the teachers with ICTs.

- Teachers are one of the key players in providing the active learning environment and driving reforms. Therefore, universities/institutions should encourage and support them to invcıve in numerous ICTs sharing sessions, training, seminars and courses.
- Universities/institutions should provide training to the teachers on how to apply and use ICTs in teaching the various concepts. Teachers should get training about the usage of floppy disc, compact disc read only memory (CD-ROM) (*X-cology* software for demonstrating the animal experiments for example), Internet (online lectures, pharmacokinetics teaching, Web based clinical trials, etc.), mobile devices (e.g., personal digital assistant (PDA)) and other information technologies (e.g., pharmacy informatics).
- In spite of initial training, teachers may need to overcome further hurdles in implementing new teaching approaches in the classrooms. New models of professional development should be developed to build in mechanisms that will encourage and support the new teaching approaches.
- Universities/institutions should use more pharmacy teaching software and indexing resources for ease of retrieval and use. There should be incentive schemes to encourage collaboration amongst colleges and relevant organizations in harnessing ICTs in teaching-learning.
- University/institution should plan for presenting a voluntary certification to recognize competencies and commitment of teachers who receive training. This motivational strategy provides extra and higher recognition for the provision of evidence and examples of how the training has led to teaching-learning changes in the classroom. A "certification

ladder" may be established with the assistance of information technology organizations as well as subject associations to encourage continuing professional development of teachers.

3) **Enhancing the leadership capacity of university/ institute for the knowledge age:** University's/ institution's heads and their associates should take guidance and support to establish ICTs-embedded visions and goals. In addition, they also should get guidance and support to build teams appropriate for the college contexts. Such teams should be enabled to effectively lead change in integrating ICTs into college planning, curricula, teaching and learning processes, communication and collaboration. Members of the teams should get more flexibility in making decisions that tailor to the needs of their colleges. This goal can be achieved by completing the following sub-goals.

   a) ***Building leadership capacities for using ICTs as a lever for curriculum innovation***

      - The university/institution leadership team needs to understand that the most important use of ICTs in curriculum is to support the curriculum reform and such technologies can be used as lever for innovation-the essence of e-leadership.
      - University/institution heads and their associates need to take professional development training/ course which will help them to understand the different dimensions of a university/institution policy and strategy (including ICTs infrastructure, curriculum goals for ICTs use, staffing policy, staff appraisal and reward policy). This training will help while implementing ICTs in the curriculum. The professional development training should be able to also provide a structure and mechanism that encourage and support university/institution

in establishing the vision, goals and strategies as well as leadership teams for ICTs development in university/institution. It is also necessary to incorporate training materials on the application of ICTs in pharmacy education into continuing professional development course for university/institution heads and their associates. The training materials may be: *1*) skills and practical advice on leading changes to use ICTs appropriately in university/institution for teaching and learning, *2*) use of ICTs to enhance the efficiency of university/institution administration, *3*) use of ICTs for university/institution-based assessment, and *4*) use of ICTs as communication tools with parents, students and other relevant parties.

- Prototypes for university/institution level policies and strategies that are associated with successful teaching-learning innovations using ICTs should be used as a main resource for e-leadership development. Structures/mechanisms should be established to facilitate the continuing collation and sharing of university/institution level prototypes of ICTs-supported university/institution change and innovation. Such a continuously evolving database of e-leadership prototypes will also serve as a professional development resource as well as a focal point for the development of a pharmacy community for institution heads.

b) ***Providing flexibility***: University/institution should be flexible to allocate resources to support pharmacy education-based ICTs plans and account for results. In other words, university/institution should reduce the restriction on use of all grants and provide the merging, thereby enlarging the scope of permissible use of the grants. Upon merging, university/

institution can have much greater autonomy and flexibility to use the grants for: *1*) employment of technical staff and support services, *2*) purchase of new software, maintenance or replacement of hardware, *3*) provision of training to teachers, and *4*) piloting new technology or organizing ICTs activities.

c) ***Getting the support***: After acquiring greater autonomy, university/institution needs to have the capacity and procedures to plan, manage and review the use of ICTs in pharmacy education. University/institution should continue to build up the capacity of the team of teachers responsible for planning and implementing ICTs in pharmacy education. University/institution should acquire support from ICTs-based industries, qualified experts and faculty on prototypes, guidance notes and role of ICTs in institution administration and management.

d) ***Maintenance and upgrading of ICTs infrastructure***: University/institution should continue to support the maintenance of ICTs hardware and systems and find ways to address the issue of existing ICTs equipments. University/institution should promote the use of "open source software" or free software, and explore viable lower cost alternatives for institutions to reduce the cost of software and lengthen the usable life of computers. University/institution should look for parents and others who can sponsor the establishment, replacement and upgrading of ICTs. Such cost sharing will help to ensure that the procurement of computers is based on institution's demonstrated need and increase the sense of ownership among the sponsors involved.

e) ***Piloting new technology***: University/institution should support and promote trial or pilot schemes to explore new technology, e.g. Internet 2. This will provide encouraging feedback. Introduce wireless technology and install common computers in university/ institution campus to remove the physical barrier of learning in classroom and promote the concept of an e-campus.

f) ***Facilitating institution's self-evaluation***: University/ institution should set-up a self-evaluation system on the effectiveness of university/institution-based ICTs plan. In this regard, a framework for benchmarking of performance and processes should be considered. The framework will help university/institution heads and management work for results by providing an accountability regime.

g) ***Facilitating university's/institution's partnership***: University/institution should encourage and facilitate forming the partnership with other universities/ institutions and the private sector. This will explore efficient ways to utilize resources and improve the use, management and maintenance of ICTs systems. In this regard, an experience and knowledge sharing platform should be established.

4) **Digital resources for learning:** University/institution should enrich the digital resources to meet the university's/institution's needs. Then, the university/ institution should conduct research on knowledge management strategies to enable resources and curriculum experiences generated from various sources (local and international), to become more easily shared, updated, retrieved, customized and utilized.

5) **Sharing and continuing professional development**

- There should be a team of practitioners and experts to conduct evaluation and research. The objective of this team is to identify effective strategies for ICTs in pharmacy education and distill the elements of successful teaching methodologies. Prototypes should be more widely shared among teachers. The team should also conduct research to establish effective models of professional development in such way that the process will not only help teachers to gain knowledge and skills, but also to provide a structure and support for continuous improvement in the application of ICTs in pharmacy education.

- To track the effectiveness of university's/institution's strategy, the concerned authority should seek resources to conduct regular surveys and longitudinal study wherever appropriate, so as to monitor and evaluate strategy implementation. Such studies will provide key suggestions for policy formulation in the future.
- University/institution needs to commission research and studies in support of the implementation of "information literacy" for students and assessment, as well as on ways to benchmark institution's ICTs in pharmacy education performance and evaluation.
- University/institution should encourage evaluation and research by tertiary institutions or college.
- The systematic evaluation, research and prototype development should be done on/considering the important components such as learning paradigms and pedagogies, teaching methodologies, education resources, university's/institution's practices, curriculum integration, systems and networks.
- Prototypes developed or identified needs to be more effectively shared among teachers. The sharing ways are: *1*) putting prototypes on web pages, *2*) sharing in sessions and seminars, and *3*) putting prototypes in resource banks or storehouses.

6) Community-wide support and community building

- The community (parents in particular) needs to be involved and encouraged to motivate students towards appropriate use of ICTs/sponsor and drive home messages on cyber ethics.

- University/institution needs to continue to encourage the private sector to support ICTs in pharmacy education.

REFERENCES

1. Apple classrooms of tomorrow project (ACOT). 1995. Changing the conversations about teaching, learning and technology: A report on 10 years of ACOT research. Apple Computer Australia Pty Ltd, Frenchs Forest, NSW.
2. Poirier TI. 2007. A new vision for pharmacy education: It is time to shift the old paradigm and move forward. American Journal of Pharmaceutical Education 71: article 103.
3. Beck DE. 2003. Where will we be tomorrow? We need a 2020 vision. American Journal of Pharmaceutical Education 66:208-210.
4. Zarotsky V, Jaresko GS. 2000. Technology in education-Where do we go from here? Journal of Pharmacy Practice XIII:373-381.
5. Maine L. 2005. Bigger, better, faster = Stronger. American Journal of Pharmaceutical Education 69: article 81.
6. Smothers V, Greenel P, Ellaway R, Detmer DE. 2008. Sharing innovation: The case for technology standards in health professions education. Medical Teacher 30:150-154.
7. Okamoto T, Cristea A, Kayama M. 2001. Future integrated learning environments with multimedia. Journal of Computer Assisted Learning 17:4-12.
8. Downes T, Perry B, Sherwood C. 1995. IT in education and teacher education in Australia. Journal of Computer Assisted Learning 11:23-34.
9. Geroski PA. 2000. Models of technology diffusion. Research Policy 29:603-625.
10. Hannafin RD, Savenye WC. 1993. Technology in the classroom: The teacher's new role and resistance to it. Educational Technology 33:26-31.
11. Means B, Olson K. 1994. The link between technology and authentic learning. Educational Leadership 51:15-18.

"I remember when all this was books......"

Chapter 9

TEACHING-LEARNING WITH INFORMATION AND COMMUNICATION TECHNOLOGIES: INTEGRATION AND EVALUATION

Kashappa Goud H. Desai

Information and communication technologies (ICTs) have proven to be potential tools for improving the efficacy of educational methods. These tools play crucial role in achieving a new vision of 2020, a vision of preparing pharmacy students for the information age, turning colleges into dynamic and interactive learning institutions and fostering collaboration among colleges, parents and the community. The success of ICTs-based educational methods is governed by the effective integration and performance evaluation of ICTs.

EVOLUTION OF EDUCATIONAL TECHNOLOGIES

When computers were commercially available, computers were used to teach computer programming. Development of the microprocessor in the early 1970s led to the introduction of affordable microcomputers into the institutions/universities at a rapid rate. As the public awareness about computers and application of technologies grew, the need for computer literacy became extremely influential and essential. In 1990s, computer communications and information access came into existence, particularly the accessibility of Internet-based services such as electronic mail and World Wide Web. Further advancements brought the information and communication based software packages, thereby stimulating the teachers to focus on the use of ICTs in teaching-learning methods.

'Technology', in its broadest term, has evolved as a solution to the problem associated with human need. Applying this theory and creating and adopting technologies, educators developed educational technology to address the educational problems. Whenever there is a perceived need in educational institutions, teachers are forced to adopt a technology. Before deciding the applications of computer technology in pharmacy education, teacher, administrator and educational system officer should ask themselves a question: what educational problem(s) needs to be addressed? In contrast, learning technology point towards the technologies that have arrived with the "information revolution" i.e. those associated with computers. In academic institutions, learning involves one or more teachers connected with a number of students, usually in a well defined physical setting. Computers, not just being the physical environment, are interactive and occupied a place within the relationship structures of the classroom and other learning environment.

INFLUENCE OF ICTs ON THE FEATURES OF TEACHING-LEARNING

The potential of ICTs in education has been well understood by the education systems and governments around the world. Various countries are investing heavily in the education system to raise the ICTs skills and prepare the students for the information society of the 21st century. Advanced tools (ICTs) have been playing a revolutionary role in the ongoing educational shift. These tools have brought transformation in the function of features of teaching-learning. Importantly, these tools have brought a shift in the role of teacher. The role of teacher is transformed from the director of learning to facilitator of the learner's direction and creator of learning opportunities. Use of advanced tools for communication, collaboration, information access and expression led to transformation of teacher-centered educational format (traditional mode) to a student-centered interactive and collaborative learning mode (see Table 9.1). However, the shift requires a significant cultural change in institutional education and mode of delivery, often using ICTs in the process of teaching-learning.

Table 9.1

The influence of ICTs on the features of teaching-learning[a]

Feature	Traditional Mode	Teaching-Learning with ICTs
Activity	Teacher centered and didactic	Student centered and interactive
Teacher's role	Fact teller and expert	Collaborator and sometimes learner
Student's role	Listener and learner	Collaborator and sometimes expert
Learning emphasis	Facts and replication	Relationship and inquiry
Concept of knowledge	Accumulation	Transformation
Demonstratior of success	Quantity	Quality
Assessment	Norm-referenced and multiple guess	Criterion-referenced and performance portfolios
Technology use	Seat work	Communication, collaboration, information access and expression

[a] **Source:** A report on 10 years of apple classrooms of tomorrow research learning-from instruction to knowledge construction, 1995, p. 13.

In ICTs-based teaching-learning mode, there are no set of strategies for a teacher. Hence, there are no set of applications of ICTs to the teaching-learning environment. However, teacher needs to balance a curriculum based instruction with inquiry and collaborative approach-based problem solving activities. The ICTs in such activities opens up opportunities to solve problems and act as tools for communication and collaboration.

INTEGRATION OF ICTs INTO TEACHING-LEARNING

To shift from the traditional teaching mode to a balanced teaching mode (balance between teacher-centered and student-centered ICTs-based educational formats), it is necessary to integrate the ICTs into the teaching-learning process. This can be achieved by creating and supporting the appropriate teaching-learning environments with ICTs. In particular, this can be done through projects using: *1*) interactive computer-based learning resources, 2) linking with networked communities of peers and experts, and *3*) online collaborations (beyond the classroom) and information access (going beyond the textbook). To move forward in the quality of teaching-learning, institutions should reform the learning activity with the use of computer and communication technologies. In this effort, critical component of the new concept is proximal learning. In proximal learning, learning takes place by the student completing the tasks for which support (scaffolding) is initially required. This support may include a teacher, peer or a technology such as the applications of ICTs. This has led to the use the term ICTs-based educational format.

In ICTs-based teaching-learning mode, teachers need to create the learning environment centered on students (students as learners) and belief that they learn more from what they do and think about rather than from what they are told. Therefore, the paramount concern in this approach is overall effectiveness of learning environment, not whether they are more effective with or without ICTs. Due to constantly evolving nature of the technology, teachers should make sure that ICTs does not overshadow the traditional teaching-learning mode. To implement ICTs support in learning, it is necessary to decide first what student, teacher or institutions wants to achieve. Then, teachers need to use long traditions of educational theory, their own experience and knowledge of the educational situation (e.g., student attributes) to make decisions about what the learning environment should look like, and what inputs into the learning process are required. Finally, by identifying the problems associated with providing learning environments and inputs, teachers need to adopt suitable ICTs-based support to provide solutions. Therefore, integration approach ends with decisions concerning ICTs support rather than starting with such decisions.

The five suggested ways to use ICTs to establish and sustain effective learning environment are: *1*) real world problems, *2*) scaffolding, *3*) feedback, reflection and guidance, *4*) local and global communities, and *5*) extending teacher learning. Hence, teachers require various kinds of technology tools at various level of student-centered learning mode. Useful tools include problem/task representation, knowledge modeling, performance support, information gathering, conversation and collaboration tools.

The above mentioned ways and ICTs tools provide theoretical framework to implement the use of ICTs to support high-quality teaching-learning environment. If students themselves can construct their own knowledge, then the role of the teacher is to provide an environment in which the learning activities support the role of the student as a learner. Then, the environment becomes learner-centered or learner-focused. Consequently, student (learner) will involve in constructing their own meaning through analyzing, synthesizing and evaluating processes, which are higher level thinking processes. ICTs are integral to the process of identifying, gathering and recording student's own learning and building the community of learners. In addition to the ICTs, teacher should consider other factors such as nature of teaching, student approaches to learning and the use of technology and access to information and resources. Then, ICTs can indeed empower the teacher with new solutions to the teaching-learning. An elevation of the importance of quality teaching-learning in education exemplifies the need for engaged, meaningful, collaborative teaching-learning mode involving challenging and real-life tasks. ICTs provide supportive dialogue, enhance interaction and help students to share and revise ideas. In particular, ICTs play crucial role in teaching-learning dimensions such as discussion (exchanging understandings), adaptation (adapting each other's ideas), interaction (engaging in interaction) and reflection (reflecting on experience).

Stages of Integration of ICTs

To integrate ICTs into the classrooms and other teaching programs, teacher must go through the following stages.

1) **Entry:** In this stage, teachers do not use the technology in the classroom and other teaching programs. Teachers rely on a specialist teacher to do it. Many educational institutions and teacher stay at this level. In this stage, one person (specialist teacher) becomes the expert and others remain as traditional teachers. For example, teacher learn the basics of using the new ICTs.
2) **Adoption:** In this stage, as per the need, teachers use one or two software applications (e.g., teacher using the Internet for preparing the lessons). But, teachers do not use the software as a part of the lesson for the students (e.g., Webquests, where students are actively involved in finding their own information).
3) **Adaptation:** In this stage, teachers begin to assign simple activities for students (e.g., typing work and peer editing). Direct instruction is the primary mode in this level. For example, teachers integrate ICTs into traditional classroom teaching-learning. Teachers often focus on increased student productivity and engagement by using word processors, spreadsheets and graphic tools.
4) **Appropriation:** In this stage, teachers use technology for making the unique things. Higher order thinking, collaborative learning and student-centered learning activities are used in this stage. Management structures begin to loosen up and student tasks are more open-ended and multi-disciplinary. For example, teachers focus on cooperative, project-based, and interdisciplinary work by incorporating the ICTs as needed.

5) **Invention:** This is the ultimate stage which shows innovation. At this level, students are engaged in learning activities that may or may not resemble traditional practices. Students have many options when approaching a new learning unit and can extend beyond the traditional boundaries placed by teacher knowledge, truly constructing their own knowledge. For example, teachers discover new uses for technology tools (e.g., designing projects that combine multiple technologies). The journey through these stages is enhanced when teachers and students have unlimited access to ICTs in the institution and look at different approaches to teaching-learning.

PRINCIPLE OF TEACHING-LEARNING WITH ICTs

ICTs-based teaching-learning is not one-sided; instead it admits a range of learning by all participants, including the teachers. To build learning communities and provide student-centered learning environment, institutions need to consider various factors. Selection of appropriate technology is one of the important factors. The selected technologies should be able to provide interactivity, learner control and student engagement. The technologies with these capabilities can improve the quality of teaching-learning. Students must be engaged in the process of learning to create an active learning environment. This can be done by motivating the students through authentic learning experiences (teaching-learning activities that should be able to demonstrate real-life connections by associating the concept of being taught with a real-life activity or event while promoting active learning).

ICTs-based teaching-learning approach can be visualized as shown in Figure 9.1. As shown in figure, the teacher brings the expertise, a syllabus or content, objectives and ICTs support to the teaching-learning environment. Teacher mediates the learning, not determines the learning. The learning in this approach is learner-focused where the learners bring prior knowledge, attitudes, skills and a variety of approaches to their own learning. Outcomes/attributes provide the vision of what the learner should achieve, critical thinking. Students are actively and meaningfully engaged in their own learning which is embedded in a social and interactive environment.

EVALUATION OF INTEGRATION OF ICTs

Teachers go through numerous concerns while integrating the ICTs into the teaching program. Upon integration of ICTs into the teaching program, one should evaluate the efficacy of implementation using an appropriate model. This can be done by addressing the concerns associated with the integration of ICTs. Several models (concerns-based adoption model (CBAM), instructional transformation model, project on the implementation of new technologies model, project information technology model etc.) have been developed to evaluate the efficacy of implementation of ICTs into the teaching program. In CBAM, teacher's concerns about innovations (ICTs) are evaluated. In particular, one would intend to study about teachers, what makes teachers use ICTs, and what makes teachers want to- or need to- use ICTs. Many models which have been developed for use in research with ICTs in the teaching program have their roots in the CBAM model. Hence, among the models developed, CBAM has been the model of choice to evaluate the effectiveness of integration of ICTs.

Concerns-Based Adoption Model (CBAM)

CBAM model consists of three dimensions (stages of concern, levels of use, and innovation configuration). The first two dimensions are explanatory and third one diagnostic in nature and scope. In other words, first two dimensions focus on the implementer while third one deals with the innovation itself. CBAM requires researchers to conduct research on each dimension and instrument to collect and present the data. The researchers should dream about innovation and constantly refine the judgments associated with the third dimension.

1) **Stages of concern:** Implementers come across numerous concerns (stages of concern) while

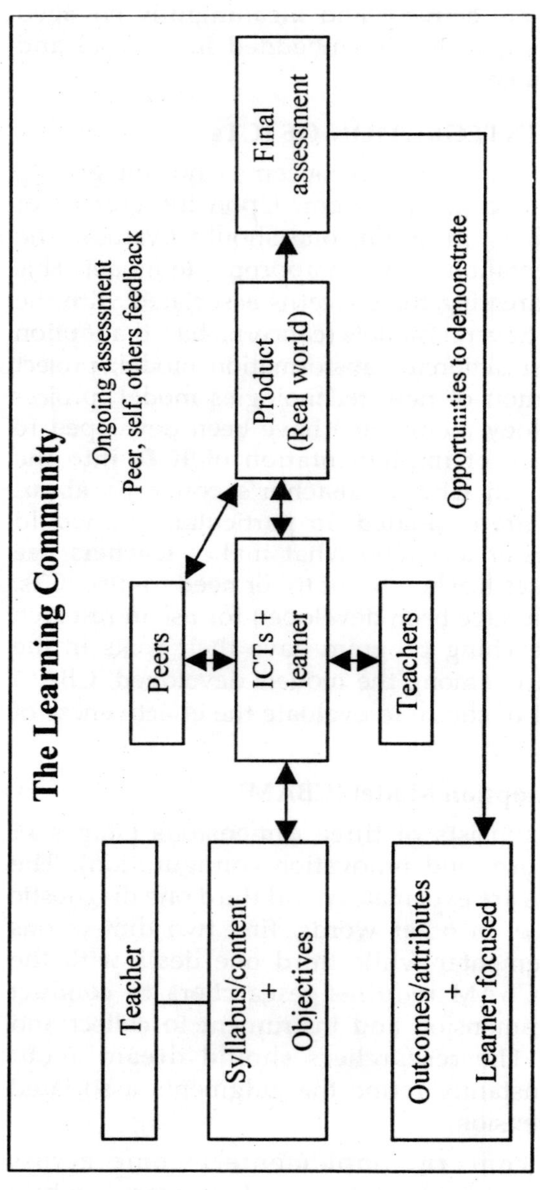

Figure 9.1. The structure of ICTs-based teaching-learning approach

implementing the ICTs in the teaching-learning program. Investigation of this dimension will tell about how teachers or others perceive an innovation and how they feel about it. Using a questionnaire (which contains scales for the type and strengths of participant's concerns), numerical and graphical picture of stages of concern can be obtained. The stages of concern, description of each stage and corresponding scale is given in Table 9.2.

2) **Levels of use:** There are various levels of technology use, from non-use to institutionalization. In this dimension, the users pass through each level as they gain in confidence and skill in using an innovation. Investigation of this dimension identifies what teacher is doing or not doing in relation to the innovation (ICTs use). This can be done by a structured interview and observations to obtain the data needed to place participants at one of these levels. The levels of technology use, description of each level and corresponding scale is given in Table 9.3.

3) **Innovation configuration:** This dimension focuses on describing the operational forms an innovation (ICTs) can take. To do this investigation, one should prepare a two dimensional chart of the innovation using existing documentation about the innovation and interviews with participants (including facilitators). In this chart, a series of statements, known as components (access to computers, student use of computers in a subject area, classroom organization, independent learning, teacher-student relationship, learning activities, nature of task environment, and technological literacy), are constructed to define the intended outcomes of the innovation. These components are listed vertically, must be able to be observed, and represent the innovation implemented fully and successfully. For each component a range of variations (1 to 4) representing status of implementation are described (see Table 9.4).

Table 9.2

Stages of concern, description of each stage and corresponding scale[a]

Scale	Stage of concern	Description of he stage
0	Awareness	Indicates little concern about or involvement with the ICTs.
I	Informational	Indicates a general awareness of the ICTs and interest in learning more detail about ICTs. At this stage, the teacher seems to be unworried about the relation between him and ICTs. But, interested in substantive aspects of the innovation in a selfless manner such as general characteristics, effects, and requirements for use.
II	Personal	Indicates that the teacher is uncertain about: *a*) demands of the innovation, *b*) inadequacy to meet those demands, *c*) role with the ICTs. This includes analysis of teacher's role in relation to the reward structure of the organization, decision making, and consideration of potential conflicts with existing structures or personal commitment. Financial or status implications of the program for self and colleagues may also be reflected.
III	Management	Indicates that the teacher's attention is focused on the processes and tasks of using the ICTs and the best use of information and resources. Highest priority is given to issues related to efficiency, organizing, managing, scheduling and time demands.
IV	Consequence	After use of ICTs, the teacher's attention is focused on impact of the ICTs on students. In particular, the focus is on relevance of ICTs for students, evaluation of student's outcomes, including performance and competencies, and changes needed to increase student's outcomes.
V	Collaboration	This stage state that the teacher is focused on coordination and cooperation with others regarding the use of ICTs.
VI	Refocusing	Indicates that the teacher is focused on exploration of more universal benefits from the ICTs, including the possibility of major changes or replacement with a more powerful alternative. Individual has definite ideas about alternatives to the proposed or existing form of the ICTs.

[a] Based on Newhouse (1998) and DEST (2001).

Table 9.3

Levels of technology use, description of each level and corresponding scale[a]

Scale	Level of use	Description of the level
0	Non-Use	The teacher has little or no knowledge of the ICTs, is not involved with the ICTs, and is not putting any efforts to become involved.
1	Orientation	At this level, the teacher: *a*) has acquired or is acquiring information about the ICTs and *b*) has explored or is exploring the value of ICTs orientation and its demands upon user and user system.
2	Preparation	This level state that the teacher is preparing for first use of the ICTs.
3	Mechanical Use	Indicates that the teacher is focused with most effort on the short-term, day-to-day use of the ICTs with little time for reflection. Teacher made more changes in usage to meet his own needs than client needs. Teacher is primarily engaged in a stepwise attempt to master the tasks required to use the ICTs, often resulting in disjointed and superficial use.
4a	Routine	Use of the ICTs is stabilized. Teacher makes few changes in ongoing use. Teacher made little preparation or gave little thought to improve ICTs use or technology's consequences.
4b	Refinement	The teacher varies the use of ICTs to increase the impact on students within immediate sphere of influence. Teacher's variations are based on knowledge of both short-term and long-term consequences for students.
5	Integration	Teacher is combining own efforts to use the ICTs with related activities of colleagues to achieve a collective impact on students within their common sphere of influence.
6	Renewal	Teacher: *a*) re-evaluates the quality of use of the ICTs, *b*) seeks major modifications of or alternatives to present technology to achieve increased impact on students, *c*) examines new developments in the field, and *d*) explores new goals for self and the system.

[a] Based on Newhouse (1998) and DEST (2001).

Table 9.4: Innovation configuration components and variations (1 to 4)[a]

1	2	3
Access to computers and technologies[b]		
All students have at all times.	All students have access at home and sometimes at institution.	Some students have computers and technologies at home.
Student use of computers and technologies in a subject area[b,4]		
Students use computers and technologies at home and in many lessons	Students use computers and technologies at home and in some lessons.	Students use computers and technologies at home.
Classroom organization[b]		
Teacher uses a variety of teaching strategies based on computer and technology use.	Teacher uses one alternative teaching strategy based on computer and technology use.	Teacher uses no alternative teaching strategies based on computer and technology use.
Independent learning[b]		
Students use computers and technologies extensively to support working at their own pace and constructing their own knowledge.	Students sometimes use computers and technologies to support working at their own pace and constructing their own knowledge.	Students never use computers and technologies to support working at their own pace and constructing their own knowledge.
Teacher-student relationship[b]		
Students do not depend on teacher for knowledge acquisition or completion of tasks on the computer.	Students often do not depend on teacher for knowledge acquisition or completion of tasks on the computer.	Students depend on teacher for knowledge acquisition or completion of tasks on the computer.

Learning activities[b]		
Students use computers and technologies to complete practical or investigative activities which are relevant to their experience. The activities will be designed to develop both higher and lower order learning skills.	Students use computers and technologies to complete practical activities which are relevant to their experience.	Students use computers and technologies to complete activities which are not always relevant to their experience but may be either practical or investigative in nature.
Nature of task environment[b]		
Students will be given tasks to complete on the computer and technology which are motivating and problem solving and students will receive regular feedback on those tasks.	Students will be given tasks to complete on the computer and technology which are motivating and students will receive regular feedback on those tasks.	Students will be given tasks to complete on the computer and technology which may be motivating but students do not receive regular feedback on those tasks.
Technological literacy[b]		
Students develop a level of technological literacy relevant to institution and entry level workplaces through the use of the computers and technologies. Students will improve the presentation of their work and use the drafting cycle.	Students develop a level of technological literacy relevant to institution through the use of the computers and technologies. Students will improve the presentation of their work and use the drafting cycle.	Students will improve the presentation of their work and use the drafting cycle.

4- 4th variation is 'students do not use computers for subject'.

[a] Based on Newhouse (1998) and DEST (2001); [b] innovation configuration component

REFERENCES

1. Apple classrooms of tomorrow project (ACOT). 1995. Changing the conversations about teaching, learning and technology: A report on 10 years of ACOT research. Apple Computer Australia Pty Ltd, Frenchs Forest, NSW.

2. Downes T, Perry B, Sherwood C. 1995. IT in education and teacher education in Australia. Journal of Computer Assisted Learning 11:23-34.

3. Means B, Olson K. 1994. The link between technology and authentic learning. Educational Leadership 51:15-18.

4. Salomon G. 1994. Differences in patterns: Studying computer enhanced learning environments. In: Vosniadou S, DeCorte E, Mandl H (Eds.). Technology-based learning environments. Springer-Verlag, Heidelberg, p. 79-88.

5. Plomp T, Pelgrum WJ. 1992. Restructuring of schools as a consequence of computers. International Journal of Educational Research 19:185-195.

6. Marcinkiewicz HR. 1994. Computers and teachers: Factors influencing computer use in the classroom. Journal of Research in Computing Education 26:220-237.

7. Lemke C, Coughlin EC. 1998. Technology in American schools: Seven dimensions for gauging progress. Milken exchange on educational technology, USA.

8. Hussein Y. 1996. The role of the computer in the school as perceived by computer using teachers and administrators. Journal of Educational Computing Research 15:137-155.

9. Newhouse CP. 1998. Teacher's responses and classroom learning environments associated with student access to portable computers. Ph.D. Thesis. Curtin University of Technology, Perth, Western Australia.

10. Department of Education, Science and Technology (DEST). 2001. Making Better Connections-Models of teacher professional development for the integration of ICT into classroom practice. Department of Education, Science and Training, Canberra.

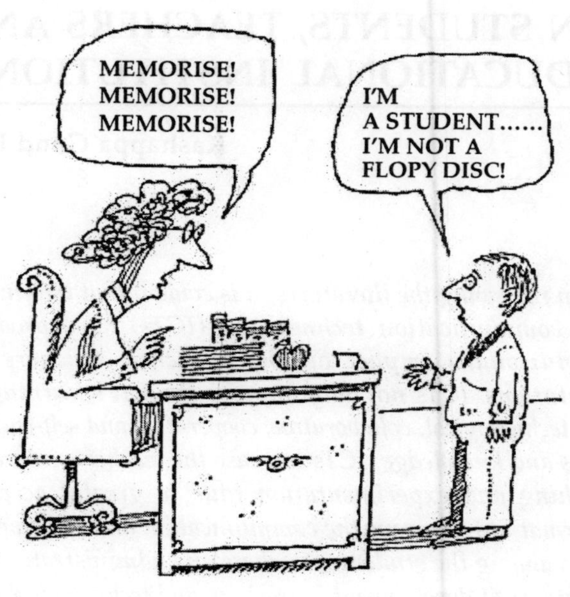
MEMORISE!
MEMORISE!
MEMORISE!
I'M
A STUDENT......
I'M NOT A
FLOPY DISC!

Chapter 10

IMPACT OF INFORMATION AND COMMUNICATION TECHNOLOGIES ON STUDENTS, TEACHERS AND EDUCATIONAL INSTITUTIONS

Kashappa Goud H. Desai

Upon reviewing the literatures, it is evident that information and communication technologies (ICTs) have produced revolutionary impact on the students, teachers and institutions. ICTs not only improve student's learning but also technological, collaborative, cooperative and self-learning skills and knowledge. ICTs increase the teacher's interest in teaching and experimentation (due to greater access to information), improve the communication and collaboration skills among the students, teachers and administrators, and facilitate self-development in teaching and technological skills. ICTs-embedded education raises the requirements in infrastructure, curriculum and technical support for teachers, institutional physical structure, organization and policies and management support. Since the educational system is continuously bombarded with constantly evolving educational technologies, advancements will continue to have revolutionary impact on students, teachers and institutions.

IMPACT OF ICTs ON STUDENTS

The needs of tomorrow's pharmacy profession are forcing the educators to adopt innovative educational technologies in teaching-learning methods. As a result, there has been drastic change in the roles and responsibilities of the students. Learning the pharmacy subjects with ICTs will stimulate/motivate the students to acquire the following skills/knowledge.

1) **Increases student's technological literacy:** The improvement in the quality of learning of various aspects of pharmacy subjects has been observed by adopting the suitable educational technology. Learning with educational technologies improves the student's technological literacy. The technological literacy is the knowledge (about systems, components, operations, capabilities and limitations), skills (in using ICTs to perform relevant tasks) and positive attitudes (toward ICTs use personally and in society) of the students they gain from learning with ICTs. Following are some examples where student's technological literacy is increased by ICTs-based learning methods.

   a) Computer-simulated (for example, Authorware Professional™ software) pharmacology experiments and pharmacokinetics studies enhances student's understandings of the subjects and computer-simulations.

   b) Learning the various complex topics (cellular parameters such as drug-receptor interactions, drug targeting, protein binding etc.) with appropriate software enhances student's understandings of the subject and associated software usage.

   c) Learning the medicinal chemistry aspects (for example, acid-base chemistry, drug design and drug's properties) with appropriate software increases student's skill in the adopted technology.

   d) Information technology (pharmacy informatics (computerized medication administration records, robots, automated pharmacy systems, bar-coding, "smart" intravenous devices, computerized discharge prescriptions and instructions)) can be used to reduce medication errors. Teaching with these technologies increases the student's technological knowledge.

2) **Empowers self-learning and professional skills:** The use of ICTs in pharmacy education empowers self-learning and useful professional skills. Unlike traditional teaching method, learning with ICTs facilitates active learning environment, thereby improving the quality of learning. Upon effective learning with ICTs, students become independent, responsible, cooperative, collaborative and directive.

3) **Engages students in educational change:** Students gain modern technological literacy from their advanced learning methods (learning with ICTs). With this cultural capital, students contribute in educational change.

4) **Increases motivation for learning:** Use of ICTs as supportive tools in learning activities motivates students for self-learning. For example, use of ICTs to introduce the topic or used for initial preparation.

5) **Improved student's achievement (score/grade) in core subjects:** Numerous studies have been conducted to test the student's preference of learning methods (traditional or learning with ICTs). After examining the student's preferences, it has been reported that students prefer modern technological methods (learning with ICTs) than traditional instruction. For example, students prefer computer-assisted learning, computer-simulated learning and learning with multi-media than traditional instruction in the study of core subjects.

IMPACT OF ICTs ON TEACHERS

Teachers play crucial role in modern technological teaching methods (teaching with ICTs). Therefore, the impact of ICTs on the teachers and strategies they employ to facilitate effective learning is critical. Teaching with ICTs requires teachers to become proficient in effective teaching, communication, technological and self-development skills. Hence, the impact on teachers is varied and characteristic. The impact of ICTs on teachers can be linked to the following areas.

1) **Roles of teachers:** Introduction of ICTs in teaching has led to the transformation in the roles of teacher. ICTs have pushed the teachers to acquire greater range of skills and understandings. Teachers have become more skilled in directing students through the huge quantities of rich information. If ICTs are used to engage students in more cross-discipline project-based learning, modern technological teaching methods facilitated teachers to have an understanding of a wider range of disciplines and learning within those disciplines. The impact of ICTs on teaching strategies has led to changes in the composition of the role of teachers. For example, high level access to computer support for learning encourages teachers to use more cooperative group work and less teacher stand-up lecturing (transformation from fact teller to facilitator of active learning). Also use of online lectures, Web-based learning and invited lectures reduced the amount of responsibility.

   Further, ICTs in education facilitated a much richer exploration of experience, but demanded a high-level of competence on the part of the teacher to facilitate students to fully benefit from this experience. As a result, teachers acquired initiative, organizing, evaluative and technological (computer-assisted teaching, computerized problem based teaching, online teaching, pharmacy informatics etc.) skills. In addition, ICTs made the teachers to be highly competent and fit for the future revolutions in the technological education.

2) **Access to information:** In the ICTs-based teaching methods, teachers sift through information efficiently. Teachers learn about collecting, organizing, processing and communicating information associated with effective

teaching. In addition, teachers adjust to diverse skills and form new attitudes. Use of ICTs provides access to information to support teachers in trying new strategies, thinking, reflecting on practice and engaging with new material. Teachers require support in making use of new educational technologies to enhance their personal work before learning to use them in their teaching. Using ICTs, much of this support can be accessed more readily.

3) **Energy, hard work and determination:** ICTs in education makes teachers to demonstrate high levels of energy, hard work and determination. If the teachers are early adopters then they become resourceful and overcome many barriers to "make things work". Implementation of ICTs provides an opportunity to develop ICTs operation and classroom management skills/knowledge in the teachers.

   There are some potential reasons for using ICTs in pharmacy education. The potential reasons are dynamic learning, student motivation, removing tedious tasks, teaching to fit the students, self-learning and extending student's thinking. Use of ICTs to fulfill each of these tasks resulted in advantageous and disadvantageous impacts. Potential reasons and associated impacts (advantageous and disadvantageous) are presented in Table 10.1. Most of the potential benefits are directed towards the student in improved learning. Very few of the benefits are directed towards the teacher's tasks in the institution. Therefore, it becomes necessary for the teachers to overcome the disadvantageous impacts (obstacles). This necessity pushes the teachers to continually work at updating their skills and knowledge in the operation and use of ICTs.

IMPACT OF ICTs ON EDUCATIONAL INSTITUTIONS

The use of ICTs in teaching-learning is taken very seriously by the educational institutions around the globe.

This revolution is in response to the increased competence among the institutions to prepare the students fit for the information age. However, every educational institution must provide vital ingredients (infrastructure, curriculum and technical support for the teachers, institutional change (organization, design, policies and practices) and support to the management) for the successful integration of ICTs in teaching-learning methods. Consequently, the need for ICTs in education makes the institutions to establish or upgrade the modern teaching-learning set-up (vital ingredients) and provides the new status for educational institutions. With the technological qualities and teacher's contribution, the institution can take the education to a new level. The educational institutions must provide the key ingredients of ICTs-based teaching-learning methods (see below).

1) **Infrastructure:** The infrastructure requirements may be viewed in terms of the electronic resources, hardware, networking, hardware organization for adequate access and implementation.

   a) ***Electronic resources***: Since the aim of ICTs-based teaching methods is to provide more student-centered learning experiences, the educational institutions must provide extensive sets of electronic resources. These resources mainly consist of data files and software applications (programs) (for example, software for pharmacokinetics, cellular parameters, drug targeting and pharmacological studies) that may be distributed online or on disc. Therefore, educational institutions need to provide teachers and students with ready and easy access to the electronic resources associated with teaching-learning.

   b) ***Hardware***: Teachers and students must get adequate access to appropriate hardware for substantial periods of time. Since the majority of programs require students to have individual access to computers, the achievement of significant results is dependent upon the amount of computer equipment available for use by the students. The ability of the teachers and students to use the computer and technologies to complete the tasks depends upon the characteristics of the computers. Therefore, the educational institutions should consider the users (teachers and students), physical setting (the layout of the classroom) and educational application while selecting the appropriate hardware.

c) *Networking*: In the current scenario, networks are more diverse in nature and consist of many computer processors, with a large variety of peripheral devices. The educational institutions need to set-up three kinds of networks including intra-institution, inter-institution and external (Internet) networks. An intra-institution network link together classrooms with the library, staffrooms and administrative area. Intra-institution network also include access to data storage devices such as compact discs and video discs, student and teacher workstations and a variety of printers. This allows teachers and students to access data in other areas of the institution without leaving their seats and teachers can transfer data and communicate with other teachers and the administration. On the other hand, inter-institution networks allow teachers and students to communicate between educational institutions, share resources and data. For example, distance education, online lectures and network teleconferencing. By using inter-institution network, groups of students can interact with a teacher or another group of students using telephones. In general, all kinds of network resources benefits students, teachers and institutions by: facilitating ICTs learning activities, giving ready access to software, allowing a variety of communications, reducing costs of equipment, increasing processing power, and facilitating the management of student learning.

d) ***Hardware organization for adequate access***: Institutions need to distribute the computers and appropriate software properly. If the institution has substantial amount of computers and appropriate software, it can establish the same throughout the institution. If institution possesses fewer computers and appropriate software, it needs to adopt following strategies.

Table 10.1

The potential reasons for using ICTs and associated impacts[a]

Potential Reason	Impact	
	Advantageous	**Disadvantageous**
Dynamic learning		• Students learn outside the teacher's own area of expertise. • Difficulty in directing and managing student learning.
Student's motivation	Managing and directing students towards the tasks becomes easy.	Students become distracted by the computer from the tasks the teacher has intended.
Removing tedious tasks	More satisfaction for teacher to direct less tedious tasks.	Some teachers prefer students to complete tedious, routine tasks as "busy" work.
Teaching to fit the students	Relieves the teacher from needing to spend a lot of time with students who need extra practice, catch-up or extension work.	
Self-learning		• Self-learning may not direct itself towards the teacher's objectives. • Additional coordination of the classroom, students and materials becomes necessary.
Extending student thinking		Student thinking goes beyond the teacher's experience or capabilities which might reduce the confidence of the teacher.

[a] Based on Becta (2002)

i. Laboratory: A group of computers and appropriate software can be made available in a central location of the institution which may be booked by a teacher. This facility can be dedicated to the classroom, part of the library or part of a learning resource centre.

ii. Mobile trolleys: A desktop computer and appropriate technology can be put on a trolley which a teacher may book and wheel into the normal classroom.

iii. Mobile laboratory: A number of reasonably portable computers (ideally notebook or palmtop size computers) and appropriate software can be made available for a teacher to book for a lesson. The computers and appropriate software are brought in and set-up for the lesson and returned at the end.

iv. Classroom computer(s): One or more computer(s) and appropriate software may be allocated permanently to a teacher's classroom.

2) **Curriculum and technical support for teachers:** Implementation of ICTs in education has been hampered by the lack of experience of teachers and the lack of consideration of appropriate educational problems to solve. Institutions need to provide appropriate technical and curriculum support for teachers to overcome these barriers (see below).

- ***Supporting users***: The computer users in institutions are students, teachers and administrators. Many teachers lack the knowledge and skills to use computers and appropriate technologies (for example, software for pharmacokinetics, drug design, cellular parameters, drug targeting, pharmacological and clinical trails studies). To use the ICTs effectively in education, teachers should have appropriate skills, knowledge and attitudes. Therefore, institution needs to provide sufficient training to the teachers. In addition, teachers need to develop skills of integrating ICTs into their teaching/learning programmes. Further, institution should facilitate professional (modern technological teaching) development programmes for teachers to maintain the skills and knowledge.

- ***Supporting implementation***: Computers and appropriate software are useful in some part of the curriculum. Computers should not be used as a general panacea to educational problems. Therefore, institutions need to buy the computers and appropriate software for specific purposes. This allows the teachers and students to make the best use of computers and software.

3) **Changes to institutions:** Educational institution needs to make/provide appropriate physical structure and policies and practices for the teachers and students to make the best use of ICTs. Following are the required changes.

- ***Physical structure***: Most of the institutions are not designed to include ICTs. Therefore, pharmacy institutions need to re-design the physical environments to include the ICTs. The physical environments changes include: *a*) rearranging the classroom, *b*) creating new spaces from old configurations, *c*) providing centralized and shared facilities, *d*) creating dedicated and flexible classroom space, *e*) developing virtual classrooms and campuses, *f*) creating learning communities through district networks, *g*) Web hosting by an external provider, *h*) classroom redesign for maximum flexibility, *i*) providing wireless technology and *j*) changing the traditional library areas.
- ***Organization of institution***: To improve the quality of teaching-learning, educational institution needs to involve more heterogeneous grouping, community organization, collaboration, interdependent

teamwork, and allow input from a range of expertise. Teachers learn to use ICTs with time and hence their own learning has implications for the ways in which they assist students to learn Therefore, institutions must encourage teachers to become partners in innovation, give time to learn and provide collegial advisers rather than supervisors.

- ***Policies and practices of institutions***: To provide rational use of all the ICTs, institutions need to have proper policies and practices for the students. Maintaining the proper policies and practices prevent misuse of the technologies, copyright concerns and legal implications. This can be done by taking student's contract for appropriate use, installing the filtering software and providing access in areas which are highly visible to staff.

4) **Support to the management:** The institutions need to use ICTs to assist in management functions. This will improve the efficiency in many of the tasks required in the operation of institutions. ICTs can be used as tools by the teacher (for course preparation, practical demonstration, student and resource management, record keeping etc.) and institution administration (for maintaining student records, managing curriculum content, supporting teaching-learning, maintaining timetables and classes, financial management, assisting communication, supporting library, communication etc.) for performing functions that are required in the running of an institution.

REFERENCES

1. Apple classrooms of tomorrow project (ACOT). 1995. Changing the conversations about teaching, learning and technology: A report on 10 years of ACOT research. Apple Computer Australia Pty Ltd, Frenchs Forest, NSW.
2. Zarotsky V, Jaresko GS. 2000. Technology in Education-Where do we go from here? Journal of Pharmacy Practice XIII:373-381.

3. Smothers V, Greenel P, Ellaway R, Detmer DE. 2008. Sharing innovation: The case for technology standards in health professions education. Medical Teacher 30:150-154.
4. Valcke M, Wever BD. 2006. Information and communication technologies in higher education: Evidence-based practices in medical education. Medical Teacher 28:40-48.
5. Furneaux C. 2004. How does information technology impact the methods, potential and purpose of education? ETL Conference, Logan Campus, Griffith University, Craig Furneaux.
6. Vogel D, Klassen J. 2001. Technology-supported learning: Status, issues and trends. Journal of Computer Assisted Learning 17:104-114.
7. Wang L. 2001. Computer-simulated pharmacology experiments for undergraduate pharmacy students: Experience from an Australian university. Indian Journal of Pharmacology 33:280-282.
8. LeBlanc PP, Aiache JM. 1994. Problem-based and computer-assisted learning of pharmacokinetics. American Journal of Pharmaceutical Education 58:94-95.
9. Roche VF, Zito SW. 1997. Computerized medicinal chemistry case studies. American Journal of Pharmaceutical Education 61:447-452.
10. Breen R, Lindsay R, Jenkins A, Smith P. 2001. The role of information and communication technologies in a university learning environment. Studies in higher education 26:95-114.
11. Rieber LP, Welliver PW. 1989. Infusing educational technology into mainstream educational computing. International Journal of Instructional Media 16:21-32.
12. Becta. 2002. The impact of information and communication technologies on pupil learning and attainment. ICT in Schools Research and Evaluation Series-7.

Chapter 11
COMPUTER ASSISTED TEACHING-LEARNING

Kashappa Goud H. Desai

"Computers can figure out all kinds of problems, except the things in the world that just don't add up"

—James Magary

Computer assisted teaching-learning (CAT-L) is a student-centered and interactive teaching-learning format in which computer(s) and simulation or software or multimedia are used as tools to teach-learn the concepts of a subject. It is inevitable, flexible and convenient, gives unique presentational benefits, offer personalized learning and expand educational horizons. Computer plays numerous roles in pharmacy education. Computer can be used to assist a lecture, provide an interactive learning environment and understand the complex topics of pharmacy subjects. Depending on the need of the study, one of the CAT-L methods (classroom learning, simulation learning, learning with software tools and multimedia learning) can be adopted.

INTRODUCTION

Pharmacy academia is taking a paradigm shift in the learning environment from the traditional teacher-centered 'teaching' to learner-centered 'learning'. Rapid expansion in the knowledge of pharmacy subjects has led to increased need for adequate approaches to teach-learn the complex topics.

In an effort to expand and improve the training of pharmacy students, educators began to use the information and communication technologies (ICTs) in the teaching methodologies. Teachers wouldn't dictate the what, how, where and when of student's learning in ICTs-based teaching-learning methodologies. Learning, then, essentially becomes a participatory outcome of learner's browsing in the learning environment singly or in a community of other learners explore together, and/or support each other, as they use information resources and tools to pursue their learning goals and solve problems. ICTs-based teaching-learning methods have revolutionized the process of education by providing self-instructions, self-evaluation, and virtualization of majority of the problems. As a result, CAT-L has become a common modality in dissipation of complex subjects.

CAT-L is a student-centered and interactive teaching-learning format in which computer and simulation or software or multimedia is used as tools to teach-learn the concepts of a subject. The first computer-assisted learning became available to the university students in the 1980s. Initially, learning programs used only digital files which then transferred onto a compact disc read-only memory (CD-ROM) to give students highly portable and accessible learning materials. The popularization of CAT-L and increased ownership of personal computers led to the development of widely distributed educational CD-ROMS. As technology continued to grow and with the introduction of the Internet, information on CAT-L programs became more interactive, reflecting a social need for flexible learning outcomes. There is now a multitude of CAT-L platforms designed for every pharmacy subject. CAT-L applications generally require the student to follow the content without immediate or direct supervision from the teacher. However, computer can be a temperamental and unforgiving beast. Therefore, CAT-L applications must embody the quality features described below.

ESSENTIAL QUALITY FEATURES OF CAT-L

1) **Open learning (self study) materials:** Computer-based study applications must be prepared in advance. The applications must include explicit course aims, learning objectives, a high degree of "signposting," explanatory text and trouble shooting information.

2) **Website design:** The designed websites should have a logical structure and sequence, utilize features such as hypertext and graphics and include links to public access Web-based materials (electronic journals where appropriate).

3) **Technical design:** Computer applications must be user friendly and operate effectively within the hardware and software constraints of the end user.

4) **University/institution culture:** Computer applications must present an academic ethos in the untidy, commercial and lenient cultures of Web-based publishing and protect the student from the distractions of the Internet.

5) **Copyright protection:** Computer applications should reflect an agreed university/institutional policy on intellectual property rights.

GENERAL ADVANTAGES OF CAT-L

1) **Inevitable:** CAT-L is inevitable. Individual lecturers and departments have already begun to introduce a wide range of computer based applications. However, some educators may use computers in a haphazard way. Therefore, planned and coordinated development is better than indiscriminate expansion.

2) **Convenient and flexible:** Use of CAT-L in courses reduces the face-to-face lectures and seminars significantly. CAT-L applications also place fewer geographical and temporal constraints on staff and students.

3) **Unique presentational benefits:** Computer presentation is an ideal choice for subjects that are visually intensive, detail oriented and difficult to conceptualize (for example, complex biochemical processes, pharmacokinetics, pharmacological process).

4) **Personalized learning:** CAT-L provides an opportunity to students to regulate their learning pace. Since each student learn the subject with a specific pace, learning process can be repeated, interrupted and resumed at student's will, which have particular advantages for weaker students.

5) **Economies of scale:** Upon the implementation of CAT-L, the incremental cost of offering it to additional students is relatively less.

6) **Competitive advantage:** CAT-L-embedded curriculum gives a new status to educational institution/university. This allows potential applicants to distinguish between pharmacy institutions. A 'leading edge' virtual campus is likely to attract good students.

7) **Achieves the ultimate goal:** Computer applications, especially the Internet and World Wide Web, efficiently link the learners into learning communities.

8) **Expands educational horizons:** Virtual campus may alter fundamentally the relation between learners and knowledge.

GENERAL DISADVANTAGES OF CAT-L

1) All topics/subjects are not suited for CAT-L.

2) CAT-L necessitates support and training for teachers and students. Without support and training, they could prove an expensive disaster.

3) Development of CAT-L requires cultural change. Some faculty and students may resist the transformation.

4) CAT-L requires careful strategic planning, resource sharing, faculty incentives, active promotion of multidisciplinary working and effective quality control. Otherwise, it will lead to ineffective implementation.
5) The process of programme development is tedious and time consuming.
6) Initial funding required to implement CAT-L is high.

TYPES OF CAT-L

Computer plays numerous roles in pharmacy education. Computer can be used to assist a lecture, provide an interactive learning environment and understand the complex topics of pharmacy subjects. Depending on the need of the study, one of the following CAT-L types can be used.

1) **Classroom learning (computers in the classroom):** Traditional lecture method, where faculty teach and student listen, has been dominating the pharmacy institution's/university's classrooms. Since traditional lecture method is a teacher-centered educational format (just listening to what teachers speak), students may not learn effectively, thereby suggesting the necessity of additional learning activities. Students need to listen, read, write and participate in classroom discussion sessions to learn through an interactive learning environment. Computer-assisted classroom teaching-learning is an effort to engage students in above mentioned activities. Briefly, selected topics are given to the students. After receiving the topic, students are expected to perform a thorough literature search (Medline or other on-line) and collect primary, secondary and tertiary references on their subject. Then, students are expected to prepare computer-based tutorial on their subject. The availability and use of computers in the classrooms provide students a new way of learning and teachers a new way of

teaching. By this approach, students will realize how useful computers are in the learning process. In addition, students will also learn about computers usage. To evaluate the effectiveness of this method, a questionnaire with a set of questions on the level of learning, personal preferences, computer literacy, faculty availability for assistance and availability of resources is prepared. Then, responses to the statements are coded and evaluated as: 1-strongly disagree; 2-disagree; 3-no feeling either way; 4-agree; and 5-strongly agree.

2) **Computer-simulation based teaching-learning:** Simulations have been found to be very useful in pharmacy education. Simulation is a computer-based technique used to imitate or simulate the interaction between a system and external stimulus. The learning process from a simulation require thorough understanding of the behavior of the simulator itself in terms of relationship between input, conceptual model and output together with the proof that an acceptable degree of confidence on the simulated results has been achieved. Simulation has been found to be a useful tool to provide convincing objective evidence of the merits of a proposed study design and analysis. Simulating a planned study offers a potentially useful tool for evaluating and understanding the consequences of different study designs. Generally, a simulation scheme entails repetitive simulation and appropriate analysis of data sets. Following are some examples of computer-simulation based teaching-learning.

   a) ***Computer-simulated pharmacokinetics study***: Pharmacokinetic simulation software (for example, Authorware Professional™ for Macintosh™) provides an additional learning tool to the students. Using appropriate hardware and the programming language or the authoring system, computer-simulated software has been developed for pharmacokinetics learning. Since the software has been developed with numerous programming languages, it does not require a teacher to elaborate programming skills. The pharmacokinetics learning software has been developed by constructing an algorithm as shown in Figure 11.1. As shown in schematic diagram, the algorithm consists of four windows: one graphical window for representing the blood concentration versus time simulations, the second, a table window, containing the values attributed to the various pharmacokinetic parameters or the physiological variables modified, the third a feedback window and the fourth a dialog window. Thus developed and used simulation scheme facilitated repetitive simulation and appropriate analysis of data sets (effect of sampling variability on parameter estimates).

b) ***Computer-simulated pharmacology experiments***: The pharmacology subject deals with the manner in which the function of living systems is affected by the chemical agents. By *in vitro* and *in vivo* animal experiments, students gain hands-on skills of pharmacological experiments and more importantly, reinforce their knowledge learned from lectures and textbooks. However, live animal experiments are time consuming, used to test a limited number of drugs at a given period of time, often labour-intensive and costly.

In the past two decades, a variety of computer-simulated programs have been developed for undergraduate and postgraduate pharmacology teaching. The computer-simulated pharmacology experiments offer numerous advantages over the traditional live animal experiments. The advantages of computer-simulated pharmacology experiments are: *a*) gives more accurate and consistent end results, *b*) offer flexibility as to when and where the experiments are conducted, and *c*) reduce the use of animals, which has been a concern of students and animal rights organizations. However, computer simulation should not totally replace the 'hands-on' experiments in the laboratory. Instead, computer simulations should be used to provide students with the opportunity to be exposed to variables in a different medium to those experienced in a real experiment. The value of such an approach can only be augmented by manipulation of simulated variables in order to generate numerical or graphical data coupled with active mental and/ or written formulation of concepts and hypotheses on the part of students.

c) ***Computer-simulated drug development***: The computer simulation has also been predominantly used in clinical trials of phase II to phase IV and occasionally applied to drug development. The need to make the drug development more efficient and informative pushed the pharmaceutical industries to make full use of the simulation technology. As a result, pharmaceutical industries, particularly the research and development personnel, are putting continuous effort to simplify and automate the drug development process using computer simulation. The pharmaceutical industry's effort has led to the development of a novel technology, computer-simulated drug development system, a method in which mathematical modeling and simulation tools are combined in an integrated environment. The computer simulations have been performed with the Trial Simulator (version 2.0) software

(Pharsight Trial Simulator, 2000). The novel system can be applied to drug development from pre-clinical studies to the first-time-in-man and the proof-of-concept studies. Computer-simulated drug development is a knowledge-based repetitive process where the newly collected information are integrated in the existing drug and disease-specific knowledge frame and used to refine and update the knowledge on the drug properties. The objective of computer-simulated drug development approach is to provide a decisional tool based on the exploration of alternative development scenarios, the evaluation of potential risks on drug

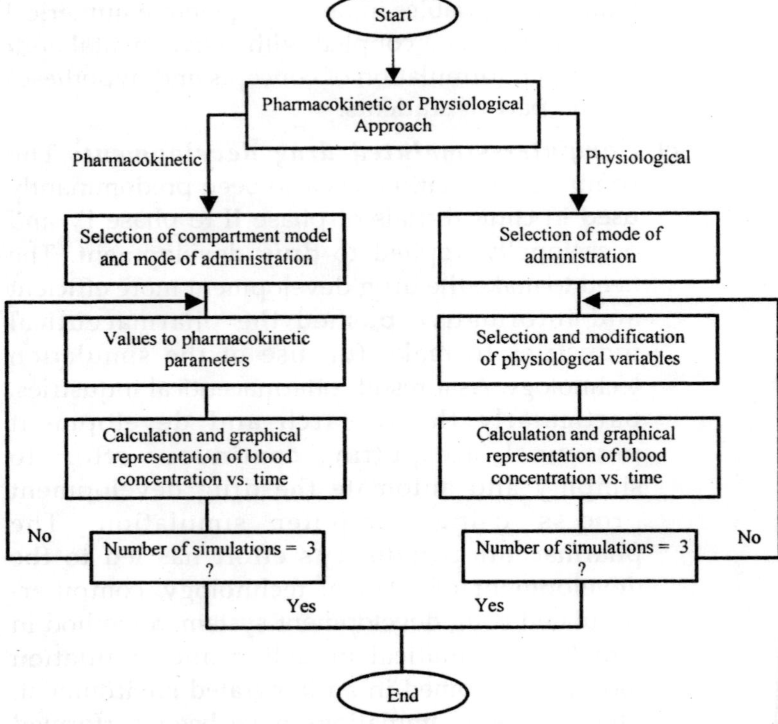

Figure 11.1. A simplified algorithm of the pharmacokinetic simulation software

safety, and the definition of experimental design of new trials with expected power and probability of success.

3) **Teaching-learning with software tools:** There has been growing demand for adequate approaches to teach-learn the complex topics of pharmacy subjects. Accordingly, easily accessible software programs have been developed for teaching-learning the complex topics of pharmacy subjects. The use of software tools in studying the complex topics makes the studies more efficient. Such software tools have been used mainly in pharmacological experiments. Following is an example of software tool used in pharmacological experiments.

   a) ***CAT-L software to demonstrate action of drug in animals***: CAT-L software programs (for example, computer assisted learning compact disc (Doerenkamp Zbinden Foundation, Germany) and Expharm ver T1.0 (Department of Pharmacology, JIPMER, Pondicherry)) have been developed for demonstrating pharmacological experiments. These software programs overcome the drawbacks (lack of ready availability of animals, higher cost of purchasing and maintaining the animals and difficulty in handling large animals like dog and cat during demonstrations in the laboratory) associated with traditional 'hands-on' experiments in the laboratory. The advantages of using software programs in demonstrating drug effects are: *a*) avoids use of animals, *b*) drug effects can be visualized clearly, *c*) exercises difficult to be conducted in the laboratory can be demonstrated using software programs, *d*) many students can observe experiments at the same time, *e*) experiments can be observed repeatedly without loss of animals and *f*) no experimental errors as observed in laboratory exercises. However, some disadvantages are associated with using software programs for demonstrating drug effects in animals. These include: *a*) experiment is programmed with prefixed doses, *b*) lack of interaction with live animals, *c*) difficult to remember the experiments, *d*) variations in response as observed in living tissue cannot be observed, *e*) requires expertise to handle problems related to computers, *f*) expensive method of teaching and *g*) practical knowledge of how to do the experiment is lost.

4) **Multimedia based teaching-learning:** Every year, a large number of animals are sacrificed to demonstrate animal experiments to undergraduate and postgraduate students. The traditional demonstrations can be humanely presented using multimedia software rather than experimental animals. The multimedia software (computer-assisted learning tool) reduces/replaces the animal use and refines the demonstrations as well the teaching process. Multimedia software acts as a tool to clearly convey the required details on animal experiments. Teaching-learning with multimedia software is a form of CAT-L in which things to be learned are organized to level-by-level or linked to each other as in a network which can be controlled by the computer. The user browses from one node of data to another. The learning process is controlled by the computer or the teacher who has planned the links (route through the nodes). The learning materials may be totally open, when every node has a link to other node, or less open with fewer links and a set route through the material. Following is an example of teaching-learning with multimedia software.

   a) Demonstrating animal experiments using multimedia software (X-cology: An interactive CD-ROM): This multimedia software has been developed in such a way that it displays complete video demonstrations of different procedures like isolation and mounting of animal tissues followed by on screen interactive interface to study the effects of various drugs on the isolated tissues. It simulates/demonstrates experiments causing undue pain to animals. The presentation is made user friendly and self explanatory. Further, the details on the experiments involving animal use are divided into different topics to facilitate their presentation and easy navigation through the details. The content of this multimedia software can be classified into following topics:

i) *The experimental animals*: In this section, biological names of the common experimental animals, animals use in experimental pharmacology and important information on the specific characteristic of each species that affects the choice of the experimental animals pertaining to particular biological activity are included.

ii) *The equipments:* The common instruments used for demonstration of animal experiments are included in this section.

iii) *Experimental techniques*: This section contains the information on manual skills and routine procedures involved in the experimental pharmacology (collection of blood samples, preparation of drug solutions and routes of drug administration).

iv) *The experimental section*: This section includes exhaustive details like video demonstrations on isolation and mounting of different tissues from experimental animals, an interactive interface to study effects of different drugs on isolated tissues, procedures to carry out bio-assays and experiments on whole animals related to screening and evaluation of drugs.

RECOMMENDATIONS FOR INTRODUCING CAT-L PROGRAM

1) **Invest in faculty development:** Developing CAT-L applications is a lengthy and skilled process. Not all the faculty can understand the technology. Therefore, faculty training should be strictly conducted on a project-by-project basis.
2) **Provide a central resource base:** Templates, modules and images developed for one study may be useful for another study within the same institution. Exchange of skills, resources and ideas between institutions must be allowed.
3) **Aim to use different methods:** Educational institutions need to prefer the CAT-L products that can be easily customized, modified, upgraded, integrated with traditional teaching material and discarded as soon as their useful life is past.
4) **Faculty incentives:** Educational institutions should give appropriate incentives and rewards to individual faculty who become active members of the virtual campus (expert in CAT-L).
5) **Multidisciplinary working:** The development and use of CAT-L in pharmacy education must involve personnel who are experts in content, teaching and technical aspects of design and delivery. A multidisciplinary team based approach is likely to be the ideal model for working.
6) **Address issues of organizational culture:** Resistance to change is most likely come from the underlying culture (values, ways of thinking, management styles and teaching paradigms) of the organization. Therefore, organization's cultural issues should be addressed through appropriate approaches.

EVALUATION OF CAT-L PROGRAM

The students should be given sufficient training and allowed to become familiarized with the computer and associated simulators or software or multimedia. At least two teachers and technicians should be present at all time. To find out the effectiveness of every CAT-L program, educators need to adopt computer-assisted as well as conventional education format for the intended subject topic (for example, conventional and computer-assisted pharmacokinetics, pharmacological experiments etc.). Then, the efficacy of CAT-L program can be evaluated by a student's questionnaire (see Table 11.1). Students need to tick one box for each question. Each questionnaire should be then evaluated on a five-point Likert scale (strongly agree; agree; no-opinion; disagree; and strongly disagree). The mean score for each question can be calculated and expressed.

Table 11.1
Student's questionnaire to evaluate the effectiveness of CAT-L program[a]

	Question	Questionnaire Designation				
		SA	A	NO	DA	SDA
1	The computer simulation/software/ multimedia of the equipment did not help me to set up the actual experiment.					
2	I have achieved my learning objectives.					
3	CAT-L program improved my understanding of the subject					
4	I would recommend this form of teaching-learning to other students or friends.					
5	I prefer CAT-L program than conventional teaching/experiments					
6	I prefer 1.5-2 hours per practice					
7	The written instructions were helpful					
8	I enjoyed using CAT-L program					
9	Overall, the simulation or software or multimedia was good/excellent					

SA = Strongly Agree; A = Agree; NO = No Opinion; DA = Disagree; SDA = Strongly Disagree
[a] Based on Wang L (2001).

REFERENCES

1. Devitt P, Palmer E. 1999. Computer-aided learning: An overvalued educational resource? Medical Education 33:136-139.

2. D'Alessandro DM, Kreiter CD, Erkonen WE, Winter RJ, Knapp HR. 1997. Longitudinal follow-up comparison of educational interventions: Multimedia textbook, traditional lecture, and printed textbook. Academic Radiology 4:719-23.
3. Okamoto T, Cristea A, Kayama M. 2001. Future integrated learning environments with multimedia. Journal of Computer Assisted Learning 17:4-12.
4. Zarotsky V, Jaresko GS. 2000. Technology in Education-Where do we go from here? Journal of Pharmacy Practice XIII:373-381.
5. Wang L. 2001. Computer-simulated pharmacology experiments for undergraduate pharmacy students: Experience from an Australian university. Indian Journal of Pharmacology 33:280-282.
6. LeBlanc PP, Aiache JM. 1994. Problem-based and computer-assisted learning of pharmacokinetics. American Journal of Pharmaceutical Education 58:94-95.
7. Gomeni R, Bani M, Angelia CD, Corsib M, Byea A. 2001. Computer-assisted drug development (CADD): An emerging technology for designing first-time-in-man and proof-of-concept studies from preclinical experiments. European Journal of Pharmaceutical Sciences 13:261-270.

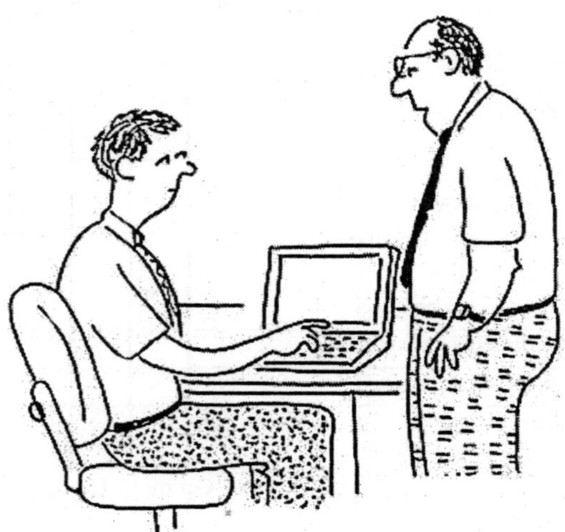

"When I was a student, wireless data transmission meant passing notes in class."

Chapter 12
WEB BASED TEACHING-LEARNING

Kashappa Goud H. Desai

World Wide Web (Web) based teaching-learning (WBT-L) is performed through a powerful, interactive and dynamic medium (Web in combination with LAN, WAN, Internet etc.) to communicate and collaborate in an educational context. It can be synchronous or asynchronous. Web has been used as an informational, supplemental, dependent and fully developed medium. Essential components of the WBT-L are: development of learning theories and educational principles, development of evolutionary software, context analysis (system scope, learning environment and stakeholders), Web and architecture design, coding and testing, and technical and educational evaluation. Electronic assessment tools, portfolio systems, individual interviews, group interviews, survey questionnaires and video-taped observation sessions are employed to evaluate the effectiveness of WBT-L. Web has been proven to be the integral part of advanced teaching-learning processes of pharmacy subjects.

INTRODUCTION

Traditional pharmacy students are more accustomed to receiving their education in the more conventional format which includes going to class, participating in class learning activities, and listening to lectures given by a teacher. However, due to time limitations, it is difficult for non-traditional students (e.g., working students or students with busy life style or students simply not being able to attend on-campus lectures due to distance) to attend on-campus learning activities/lectures. Therefore, non-traditional students prefer non-traditional methods of teaching than traditional teaching. As an effort to provide greater convenience and flexibility to the non-traditional students (learners), pharmacy education is now going through a transformation phase where the traditional, centralized, local, classroom environment is being transformed to a decentralized, distant, and virtual classroom with the help of information and communication technologies (ICTs). By using personal computers and Web-based programs effectively, flexible teaching-learning method (WBT-L) has been introduced.

WBT-L is an advanced technological approach to teaching-learning that utilizes a powerful, interactive and dynamic medium (Web in combination with local area network (LAN), wide area network (WAN), Internet etc.) to communicate and collaborate in an educational context. It can be synchronous (teacher-facilitated) or asynchronous (self-directed, self-paced). Teaching can be performed by a combination of static methods (learning portals, hyperlinked pages, screen cam tutorials, streaming audio/video, and live Web broadcasts) and interactive methods (threaded discussions, chats and desk-top video conferencing). Web-based teaching-learning entails content in a Web browser (not just activities) and actual learning materials delivered in Web format. Web browsing the learning content (even linearly) is the key feature of WBT-L. Web-based learning content is typically retrieved from a Web site, but alternative solutions are acceptable (a hypertext Web does not require Internet or networks). For instance, some WBT-L offerings operate from compact disc read-only memory (CD-ROM) and many are offered on dual format: Web site and CD-ROM.

FEATURES OF WEB-BASED COURSE

1) Course information, notice board and timetable.
2) Curriculum map.

3) Teaching materials (slides, handouts and articles).
4) Communication via email and discussion boards.
5) Formative and summative assessments.
6) Student management tools (records, statistics and student tracking).
7) Links to useful internal and external Web sites (for example, library, online databases and journals).

ADVANTAGES OF WBT-L

1) This method has the ability to link learning resources in many different formats.
2) Delivery of course materials can be done efficiently.
3) Access to learning resources is available anytime, anywhere, around the globe.
4) It is a potential method for widening access. For example, to part time, mature, or work based students.
5) It encourages more independent and active learning.
6) It provides a useful source of supplementary materials to conventional programmes.
7) The cost of set-up is relatively low. Per-student equipment costs are affordable.
8) Students complete their learning/training while they are connected to the network. Therefore, this method provides an easy student-tracking system. Unlike with CD-ROMs that require students to print reports or save scores to disk, WBT-L enables the data to be automatically tracked on the server-computer.
9) There is virtually no storage limitation and content can be held on one or more servers. The best Web-based learning is designed so that content is 'chunked' into discrete knowledge objects to provide greater flexibility. Students can access these objects through pre-defined learning paths, use skill assessments to generate personal study plans or

employ search engines to find exact topics. Therefore, possible 'learning object' architecture supports on demand, personalized learning.

10) Learning content can be easily updated. This is perhaps the single biggest benefit to WBT-L.

DISADVANTAGES OF WBT-L

1) Access to appropriate computer equipment can be a problem for students.
2) Students find it frustrating if they cannot access graphics, images and video clips because of poor equipment.
3) The necessary infrastructure must be available and affordable.
4) Information can vary in quality and accuracy, so guidance and signposting is needed.
5) Students may feel isolated.

WEB APPLICATIONS

In a course, Web can be used in four different ways. These are: informational, supplemental, dependent and fully developed use.

1) **Informational use:** In this application, course information (course outline and assignment descriptions) is made available on the Web.
2) **Supplemental use:** Students use the Web to complete part of the course. The learning materials generally include links to the related secondary sources.
3) **Dependent use:** Most learning materials already exist on the Web and students (partly) use the Web to complete the course assignments.
4) **Fully developed use:** In this application, the entire course is delivered via the Web. This is deemed as offering the course totally online without the students and teachers meeting face-to-face.

DESIGN OF WEB-BASED TEACHING-LEARNING SYSTEM

The success of WBT-L is mainly governed by the design of WBT-L system. The WBT-L activities can be performed effectively only when the system is designed adhering to the learning paradigm and associated educational principles, and to the factors that constantly affect the development of WBT-L. Therefore, one would adopt a disciplined and systematic approach to the development process for incorporating and translating the specific requirements of WBT-L into a system that constantly evolve in order to ensure the relevance, correctness and completeness of the content available on the Web. Appropriate WBT-L system has been developed by considering and completing the following essential components/requirements.

1) **Learning theories and educational principles:** Appropriate learning theory is an educational foundation upon which any WBT-L system is designed. Although there are many contemporary learning theories, not a single theory is widely accepted. However, based on the literature, available learning theories can be related to three main commonly accepted paradigms: *a*) behaviorism, *b*) cognitive constructivism, and *c*) social constructivism. The behaviorist paradigm assumes the existence of objective knowledge independent of the learners (students) whereas the cognitive and social constructivist paradigms view knowledge as a constructed entity made by each learner (student) and group of learners (students) through a learning process. Therefore, based on the objective of learning, appropriate learning theory/theories is/are adopted to develop a WBT-L system.

2) **Evolutionary software development methodology:** Education and state of the art in educational technologies are being evolved constantly. In

addition, the changes are being inflicted by academic institutions, course content and the subject domain. Any changes in the above mentioned aspects of education influences the software development process of WBT-L. Thus, WBT-L systems are developed in such a format that they constantly evolve in order to meet their requirements. WBT-L systems deal with change and evolution. The development process and associated modeling languages, techniques and tools provide support for evolution and change. A rigorous, but flexible, development methodology is adopted for WBT-L in order to avoid faulty solutions, poor quality, bad analysis, design and maintainability.

3) **Management and development process:** An evolutionary process model for WBT-L encompasses two types of processes: project management process and development process. The project management process is concerned with project planning activities that are required to manage the development process. The objective of project planning is to provide a framework that enables the project manager to make estimates of resources, costs, risks and schedule. These estimates are made within a limited time frame at the beginning of the project and are updated as the project progresses. The development process is related to a software life cycle that is required to produce WBT-L. An object-oriented software lifecycle is an orderly set of activities conducted and managed for each project. The lifecycle identifies the phases along with the software product moves from the analysis of the context to delivery and evaluation as listed below.

A) Context analysis

1) *System scope and learning environment*: The system scope ensures that the requested changes do not go beyond the accepted scope. The system scope

is determined through the identification of the learning environment that directly influences WBT-L. The environment can be characterized as the context of the system, which can best be described with six dimensions: the course content, learner, legal, ethical, technical, educational and usability issues.

2) *Stakeholders*: Variety of different kinds of people who have direct or indirect influence on the system requirements are learners/students, content developers, educational researchers, Web developers, graphic designers and Web administrators.

B) *Requirements definition and specification*: The requirements definition and specification phase captures systems requirements and defines them as natural language statements with uniform resource locator (UML) diagrams. The requirements definition and specification is concerned with technical usability criteria, educational usability criteria, system requirements and system constraints.

C) *Design*: The design phase is concerned with Web design and architecture design.

1) *Web design*: The structure of the Web is hierarchical with the top as the home page which presents general information about the system. The system is broken down into smaller components, which themselves may consist of one or many Web pages according to the topics and sub-topics of the subject matter.

2) *Architecture design*: Architecture design is done in terms of the software/hardware platform on which the WBT-L system is going to be implemented. This platform is the three-tier client/server architecture that separates data management (entity) from presentation (boundary) via the

application logic middle tier (control).

D) ***Coding and testing***: In this phase, multimedia elements (e.g. text, graphic), animation and audio which are associated with the WBT-L are produced. This is followed by the implementation of the study material associated with the content pages using programming languages or specialized authoring systems or tools such as FrontPage or Macromedia Dreamweaver.

E) ***Technical and educational evaluation***: The evaluation is necessary to ensure that the objectives are kept in mind and that the decisions made throughout the phases are achieved. Assessment of educational value of WBT-L is performed using the evaluation instruments. For example, individual interviews, group interviews, survey questionnaires and video-taped observation sessions are relevant instruments to obtain the data on what learners feel and think about WBT-L. Students/learners examinations and test performances are also used for assessing the effectiveness of WBT-L for acquiring skills and knowledge of the subject matter. Finally, teacher reflections and expert opinions in educational research are also good instruments to elicit the educational value of WBT-L. After the evaluation, the system may eventually be changed, updated and improved according to the recommendations expressed by the evaluation team.

ROLES OF TEACHER

The principle role of a teacher is to act as a 'facilitator of learning' and ensure that the educational process occurs amongst the learners (students) involved. In particular, provide guidance and allow students to explore the course materials as well as related materials without restriction. As a facilitator, teacher should perform educational (revolving around educational facilitation), social (creating a friendly social environment that is needed in the process of WBT-L), managerial (setting agendas, objectives, rules and decision making norms) and technical (teacher's proficiency with the use of the technology) tasks effectively.

ROLES OF STUDENTS (LEARNERS)

Students must be active and their roles extend to knowledge generation, collaboration and process management.

1) **Knowledge generation:** Students must actively seek solutions to the problems confined in the topic/ subject being studied with guidance from the facilitator. Students must also reflect on problems and questions presented by the facilitator and/or other students.

2) **Collaboration:** Since it (WBT-L) is a collaborative and cooperative based learning approach, students should work together to gain deeper level of understanding of the course material. In addition, students must share their resources and other learning materials with other students.

3) **Process management:** Students must participate in learning process with minimal guidelines, interact with one another and speak up when the discussions are moving into an uncomfortable zone. Also, students must speak out when they are offended and voice their opinion.

EVALUATION OF WBT-L PROGRAM

The evaluation of WBT-L environment depends highly on the evaluation instruments used and position of the evaluation in the design cycle. Evaluation can be summative or formative. To obtain data on what learners feel and think about WBT-L, assessment methods such as individual interviews, group interviews, survey questionnaires and video-taped observation sessions are employed. Numerous assessment tools or portfolio systems have also been developed. Following is a popular electronic evaluation tool which consists of multidisciplinary evaluation parameters.

Multidisciplinary framework evaluation tool: The evaluation process consist of educational and system usability sections. Since the evaluation process is quite laborious (teachers, engineers, experts etc.), an evaluation tool based on multidisciplinary evaluation framework of WBT-L is employed. WBT-L environment is being evaluated from various points-of-view to improve the quality of it constantly. In this evaluation framework, key parameters of WBT-L environment such as usefulness (see below for variety of usefulness parameters), accessibility (design of the Web should be such that the posted information should be easily accessible to all persons) and informational quality (the information on the Web should meet five main criteria: accuracy, authority, objectivity, currency and coverage) are evaluated. Responses to all evaluative parameters are collected online and stored in a server/hard drive. Following are the variety of usefulness parameters.

1) Usability
   a) Easy to learn
   b) Efficient to use
   c) Easy to remember
   d) Few errors
   e) Subjectively pleasing
2) Utility
   a) Value added
   i) Organization of teaching process
   ii) Development of quality of teaching
   iii) Development of student's learning skills
   iv) Testing and development of educational ICTs

b) Educational usability

i) Support for organization of teaching and studying

ii) Support for learning and tutoring processes as well as achievement of learning objectives

iii) Support for the development of learning skills

EXAMPLES OF WBT-L

Based on the course/subject topic, appropriate WBT-L systems have been designed and implemented in the pharmacy education curriculum. The steps involved in the design and evaluation of WBT-L program in pharmacy curriculum is similar to as described in previous sections. Web has been used as a fully developed WBT-L medium or supplemental to the traditional teaching. An example which belongs to each category of use is described below.

1) **Virtual-Recitation-A Web-based approach to active learning in clinical pharmacokinetics:** This is an example of fully developed WBT-L medium. An online computerized recitation system (Virtual-recitation) has been developed. The system allowed students to complete the assignments when it was convenient to their schedules. The virtual-recitation program was described to the students on the first day of class. Students accessed the pages via the Web through the university computing services using their computer accounts on campus or by dial-up from off campus using a Web browser in each case.

   Hypertext mark-up language (HTML) programs were used to design and post Web pages. All lectures of the course were conducted with a course coordinator. The course coordinator, using the technology, posted a series of Web pages of each week's progress that generally: *a*) summarized the important points of the week's lecture, *b*) provided clinical patient-related examples of the concepts covered in class, *c*) included two or three clinical problems for the student to solve and *d*) contained a brief formative quiz over the material that students completed on-line and submitted using 'forms' technology of the Web.

Answers to the exercises, questions to the instructor, details of discussion on topics related to course material, and information distribution (office hours, grades, exams, etc.) were posted on the Web pages. The selected software automated much of the programming generally required in Web page authoring. The program generated a Web page that contained a form (containing both multiple choice and text-box responses) which was then 'filled-out' by the online users. Responses to the form (quiz answers in this case) were sent via e-mail. The program scanned incoming e-mail for responses, which were collected into the program's database.

The objectives of implementing WBT-L component in an advanced clinical pharmacokinetics course were: *a*) to increase the student's understanding of clinical pharmacokinetics through the innovative use of active learning and available computer technologies, *b*) to increase the information and computer literacy skills of the students through hands-on computer use, and *c*) to increase the student's critical thinking and problem solving skills. The WBT-L course was evaluated by a survey of the student's opinions of the course. Students gave favorable response to the questionnaire. The Web based course improved the student's understanding of clinical pharmacokinetics through the active learning environment created by the WBT-L system.

2) **Web-based lecture notes and conferencing for an on-campus course in nonprescription drugs (Doctor of**

Pharmacy (PharmD) curriculum): In this case, the Web has been used as a supplemental to the traditional educational format (lecture). The Web page for the course has been designed based on a template. Online course design consist frames (frames divide a browser's window into separate areas, each of which can display a separate, scrollable page). A navigation frame guides the students and takes through the essential components of WBT-L system (description of the course, grading policies for the course, a list of instructors, the syllabus, current news about the course, online lecture notes, practice quizzes and conferencing).

Three live lectures were given per week. Students were then provided with supplemental online lecture notes that included text, images and hyperlinks that could be accessed at any time. In addition, students were asked to complete assignments and submit them to the instructor utilizing conferencing software. Online practice quizzes were also made available to the students for self-assessment.

In the above mentioned course, the objectives of using Web technology as a supplemental to the traditional educational format were to: *a*) encourage students to explore course topics using Internet resources, *b*) provide convenient and ready access to course faculty, *c*) provide the students with text, images and hyperlinks to additional information that the student could access whenever was convenient, *d*) take quizzes and complete assignments online using conferencing software, and *e*) evaluate student outcomes and satisfaction. It was anticipated that the inclusion of Web technology to the course would furnish a mechanism to provide continuous learning after class and foster continued dialogue about course topics between faculty and students. The efficacy of supplemental Web technology in the traditional educational course was assessed using a survey instrument. The survey instrument contained numerous survey questions on the course elements. Not surprisingly, with the help of Web-based software, the students learned more about course topics and course satisfaction could be increased. Further, students had more interaction with the course faculty than in a normal class that did not utilize conferencing software.

REFERENCES

1. Wolfe TA, Carnes CA. 1999. Comparison of Web-based and classroom instruction within a PharmD therapeutics course. Journal of Pharmacy Technology 7:59-67.
2. Goram A. 1999. The World Wide Web: An effective adjunct in clinical pharmacy skills education. Clinical Research and Regulatory Affairs 16:183-192.
3. Schewe K-D, Thalheim B, Binemann-Zdanowicz A, Kaschek R, Kuss T, Tschiedel B. A 2005. Conceptual view of Web-based e-learning systems. Education and Information Technologies 10:81-108.
4. Woodward DK. 1998. Virtual-recitation: A World Wide Web based approach to active learning in clinical pharmacokinetics. American Journal of Pharmaceutical Education 62:329-332.
5. Pruchnicki MC, Bennett MS, Legg JE, Mungall D. 2005. Development and implementation of a Web-based advanced teaching experience. American Journal of Pharmaceutical Education 69:143-151.
6. Hedayal MA, Collins C. 1999. Pharmacokinetic teaching utilizing the World Wide Web: A flashlight™ assessment. American Journal of Pharmaceutical Education 63: 415-421.
7. Engle JP, Parent-Stevens L. 1999. Developing Web-based lecture notes and conferencing for an on-campus course in nonprescription drugs. American Journal of Pharmaceutical Education 63:421-426.
8. Chang C-C. 2001. Construction and evaluation of a Web-based learning portfolio system: An electronic assessment tool. Innovations in Education and Teaching International 38:144-155.

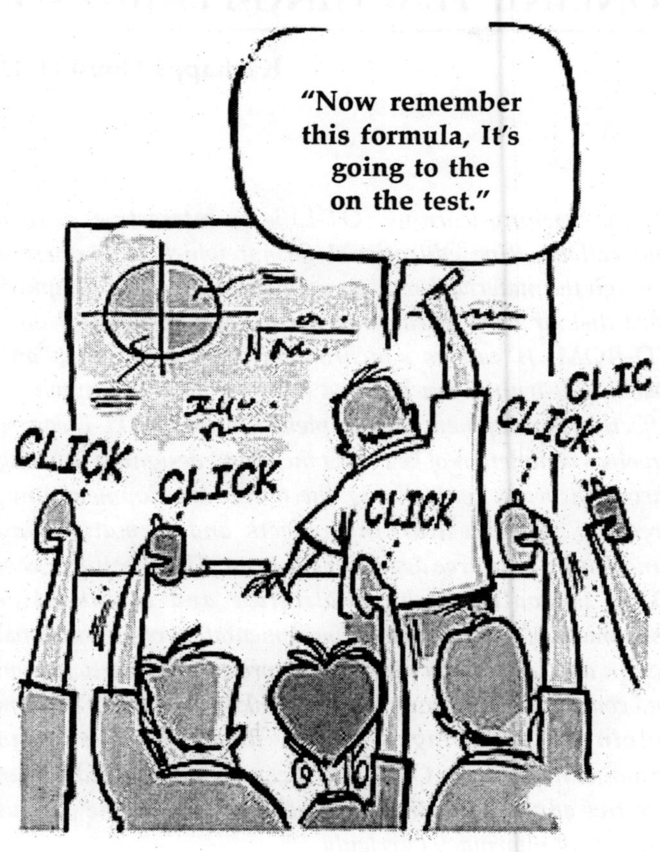
"Now remember
this formula, It's
going to the
on the test."
CLICK
CLICK
CLICK
CLICK
CLIC

Chapter 13
ONLINE TEACHING-LEARNING

Kashappa Goud H. Desai

Online teaching-learning (OT-L) is an interactive, flexible and collaborative educational format which is performed through the materials/content readily accessible on a computer hard disk or Web or the Internet or simply installed on a CD-ROM. It can be synchronous or asynchronous and teaching-learning can be done at any time and anywhere. Effective development and implementation of OT-L course involves completion of key tasks including designing learning theory/theories, centralizing the online development unit, creating reusable learning objects and formation and functioning of course development team. The effectiveness of OT-L is evaluated by qualitative and quantitative assessment of OT-L domains (implementation of instructional design and technology use, student preferences, participation and contribution, learning, critical thinking and group problem solving, advantages and disadvantages and recommendations). OT-L has been demonstrated as an effective advanced method for teaching-learning the various subjects of pharmacy curricula.

INTRODUCTION

Pharmacy education has been significantly influenced by the advent of the information and communication technologies (ICTs). With the help of computer, Internet and World Wide

Web (Web), learning has become increasingly available 'online'. Internet facilitates student-centered learning environment, thereby tailoring the education to the needs and abilities of individual students, and making life-long learning a practical reality for all. Web-based education can be provided: in places where there is none, where resources are scarce, at anytime and anywhere, for all students. Web-based education connects people, communities, and resources and can provide multiple pathways for learning to suit the needs of a diverse group of learners. A notable shortcoming is that Web-based education can worsen the divide between those who have access to online learning and those who do not. Therefore, to provide greater flexibility for learners, OT-L has been introduced.

OT-L is associated with learning materials/content readily accessible on a computer hard disk or Web or the Internet or simply installed on a compact disc read-only memory (CD-ROM). Online learning is related to the more common concepts of online help, documentation, and services. However, if learning materials are available online on a network and readily accessible, the process also qualifies as OT-L. Compared to Web-based teaching-learning (Web in combination with local area network (LAN), wide area network (WAN) and Internet), network use is not necessarily required for OT-L. In fact, the concept of OT-L surfaced before the development of 'Web' and learning materials were delivered over the Internet or networks. Web-based teaching-learning and learning courseware accessible from within a core application also often qualifies as OT-L. However, having to search for or open a separate application to access learning materials does not qualify as OT-L since the materials are not readily accessible. Neither placing information on the Web nor linking to other digital resources on the Web constitutes OT-L. OT-L occurs when students use the Web to go through the sequence of instruction to complete the learning activities and achieve learning outcomes and objectives.

Research about the size and scope of OT-L has been conducted and found that it is not clear-cut. Due to difference in learning and technologies aspects, definitional issues arose. OT-L is often combined with other approaches, making it difficult to isolate and measure. In fact, pure online teaching-learning would rarely be the mode of first choice for students and generally be used only when other approaches are not readily available. Students prefer hybrid approaches which mix modes of delivery, resources and technologies to achieve maximum flexibility and interaction with both teaching staff and their fellow students. In this way, the learning processes accommodate a range of preferred learning styles. Online technologies are used to facilitate contact and communication between teaching staff and students and students themselves. They are also used to introduce an element of face-to-face communication or improve interaction where classroom delivery is impossible or difficult. Good communication is one of the key features students look for in a teaching program.

BENEFITS OF OT-L

For Students

1) Learning can be done at any time and anywhere.
2) In asynchronous OT-L, students can access the online materials anytime.
3) Synchronous OT-L allows for real-time interaction between students and instructors.
4) Students (learners) can use the Internet to access up-to-date and relevant learning materials, and can communicate with experts in the field which they are studying.
5) Situated learning or the application of knowledge and skills in specific contexts is facilitated since learners can complete online courses while working on the job or in their own space, and contextualize the learning.

For Teachers

1) Tutoring can be done anytime and anywhere.
2) Online materials can be updated and students can see the changes immediately.
3) When students are able to access materials on the Internet, it is easier for instructors to direct them to appropriate information based on their needs.
4) If designed properly, OT-L systems can be used to determine student's needs and current level of expertise. Further, OT-L system can be used to assign appropriate materials for students to select from to achieve their desired learning outcomes.

FEATURES OF HIGH-QUALITY ONLINE TEACHING-LEARNING

Students, teachers, online material and learning assessment methods should qualify the essential characteristics to conduct the high-quality OT-L. One of the research groups has identified a range of essential features responsible for the high-quality OT-L. The essential features of OT-L have been identified based on the student's (Figure 13.1) and teacher's point-of-view. The essential features of high-quality OT-L identified based on the teacher's point-of-view are listed below.

1) Student support needs
   a) Pre-enrolment support
   b) Teaching and learning support
   c) Technical support
2) Teachers support needs
   a) Recognition by management of the need to support online teaching staff, taking into account management structures, casualisation of the teaching workforce, as well as changes related to new course content, learning resources and technology

b) Training in use of new technologies to ensure effective communication and interaction

c) Dealing with technology problems

d) Writing and other communication skills involved in using the online medium

e) Conducting assessment online

f) Market research skills

g) Skills in evaluating the effectiveness of learning experience provided online

h) Skills to facilitate the development, maintenance and improvement of online programs and resources

3) Professional development needs

a) Reflecting on pedagogical issues

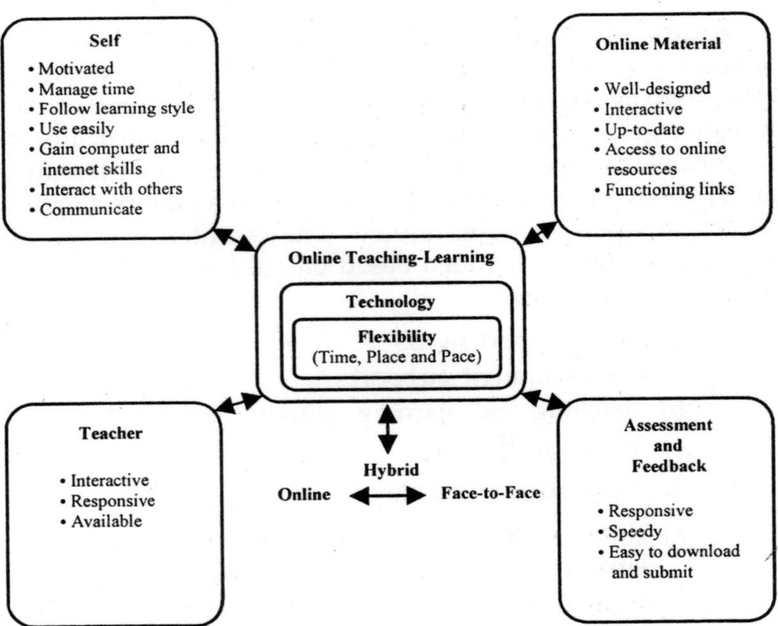

Figure 13.1. Essential features of high-quality OT-L: The learner (student's) view

   b) Using the technologies
   c) Seeing what others are doing
   d) Keeping up-to-date with new developments in a fast-moving field
   e) Resource development
   f) The development of adequate levels of written and other communication skills for the online environment
4) Accessing online
   a) Valid
   b) Reliable
   c) Flexible
   d) Fair

ONLINE COURSE DEVELOPMENT

Online course development is a complex process. It requires a highly organized and concerted effort from personnel of relevant areas. The design of online course is very similar to the design of web-based teaching-learning system (see Web-based teaching-learning chapter). Following are the stages/steps that are completed to develop an effective online course.

1) **Learning theories and educational principles:** The goal of OT-L approach is to promote active learning at anytime and anywhere. Since the teachers and students work separately, the online course developers first decide about the principles of learning and how students learn. The development of effective OT-L materials is based on proven and sound learning theories. To know about learning theories, please refer the Web-based teaching-learning chapter.
2) **Centralize the online development unit:** Developing high-quality courses and meeting institutional

guidelines are fulfilled by centralizing Web development roles into one departmental unit. Roles in this group include project manager, copy editor, information technology expert, hyper text markup language (HTML) and extensible markup language (XML) coder, media developer, instructional designer, graphic designer, administrative assistant and sometimes copyright officer.

3) **Reusable learning objects:** Repositories of reusable learning objects are created. This allows educators to submit, use or exchange the learning objects. Some examples of successful repositories are Merlot, education network Australia (EDNA) and science, mathematics, engineering and technology education (SMETE) digital library.

4) **Formation and functioning of course development team:** The core of an online course development team comprises of five key roles: subject matter expert or author, graphic designer, Web developer, programmer and instructional designer.

   a) *Subject matter expert*: Subject matter expert (SME) performs the following functions.

   - SME ensure that the content of the online course is an appropriate alternative to the lecture content normally given in a traditional course.
   - SME write the exercises, activities and examinations needed to reinforce the new learning.
   - SME work as an integral part of the team throughout the development process, ensuring that the online course content is easy to access and interesting for students.
   - SME identify or create textbooks, readings and resources.

- SME ensure an educational match among the course objectives, content, exercises, examinations and assignments.
- SME identify materials that require copyright clearance and provide the instructional designer with the necessary information.
- SME provide other team members with a legible copy of any written material.

b) *Instructional designer*: Instructional processes are analysis (the process of defining what is to be learned), design (the process of specifying how learning will occur), development (the process of authoring and producing the materials), implementation (the process of installing the instruction in the real world) and evaluation (the process of determining the impact of instruction). Instructional designer complete the above mentioned processes.

c) *Web developer*: Web developer performs the following roles.

- Web developer shows examples of online materials (which illustrate various kinds of content and interactive options) to the faculty.
- Web developer describe to faculty how their courses can be produced using a consistent organizational template that provides students with knowledge of the learning objectives, an outline of the content, assignments, evaluation information, resources, links, a list of requirements and frequently asked questions (FAQs).
- Web developer helps the SME or instructor to use tools to create the course Web pages, and to maintain the course when complete.

- Web developer helps the instructor or tutor to use the tools needed (e.g., email and chat utilities to make the course interactive).
- Web developer works with the graphic designer to conceptualize the screens, backgrounds, buttons, window frames and text elements in the program.
- Web developer creates interactivity and determine the look and feel of the interface.
- Web developer creates the design of story-boards.

d) *Graphic (Visual) designer*: Learning in OT-L method is enhanced by including technical drawings, illustrations, graphics and photography to interpret course content. Visual design includes the development and creation of generic or customized templates, navigational icons, icons or images to aid recognition of location within a non-linear presentation of materials, and visuals or graphics to enhance textual content.

e) *Programmer and multimedia author*: The programmer is responsible for program functionality. The programmer uses specialized software tools to enable the interactivity that is suggested and desired in online courses.

EVALUATION OF OT-L

The evaluation of OT-L program is performed on the basis of seven domains (see Table 13.1). Based on the objective (domain), the assessment (qualitative or quantitative) method is determined. The OT-L domains and qualitative and quantitative evaluation parameters are listed in Table 13.1.

EXAMPLES OF OT-L

1) **Online PharmD (Doctor of Pharmacy) program for pharmacy practitioners:** In this program, self-study,

Table 13.1

Evaluation strategies of OT-L program[a]

Evaluation Domains	**Quantitative Evaluation**	**Qualitative Evaluation**
Implementation of instructional design and technology use		Criteria validity by checked expert teachers
Student preferences	Multiple-choice questions	
Participation and contribution	Score based on criteria	
Learning	Post-test scores	Content analysis of discussion
Critical thinking and group problem solving		Thematic analysis of open-ended question responses
Advantages and disadvantages		Content analysis of open-ended question responses
Recommendations		Content analysis of open-ended question responses

[a] Based on the Mahoney et al.

readings, case (standard and site-specific case)-based assignments, and synchronous online chats session were utilized as OT-L strategies. The study group employed First Class® Intranet client software (SoftArc Inc. First Class®). This software is a secured integrative e-mail system and allowed interactive keyboard chat and exchange of information. Posting of documents on the Web was performed either by the teacher or the student. Generally, a one-credit module includes two chat sessions (two hours/each), four case-based assignments and self-study material. A pre-test of knowledge was conducted upon entry into the program. Frequency of activities such as obtaining patient medication history, screening for drug-related problems and care planning was assessed by a survey of participants. A ranked score was assigned to the responses given by the participants.

Changes in baseline and follow-up survey scores of pharmaceutical care activities and perceived preparedness were evaluated. Participants were asked to complete course evaluations. Statements to assess the student's perceptions of online teaching were included in this evaluation. These tasks were completed online utilizing Web course tools (WebCT). The goals of this program were to develop an online PharmD program that prepares practitioners with background and skills to provide pharmaceutical care and conduct a preliminary evaluation of the impact of the program on the knowledge of participants, frequency of pharmaceutical care activities and their perceived preparedness to provide pharmaceutical care. Not surprisingly, participants felt that the online program facilitated more active and enhanced learning environment and met their needs as adult distance learners.

2) **On-line module for teaching bayesian forecasting principles in a clinical pharmacokinetics:** A Web-based module has been developed as a learning tool for pharmacokinetic parameters estimation based on non-linear regression analysis and bayesian principles. Microsoft Excel® Solver was used to perform the bayesian analysis. A database acted as a bridge between the client's Web browser and the Excel® program. The user inputs the data into a table in the Web browser and the database relays the input to the Excel® program and sends the output of Excel® back to the user. Users access the Web page, enter an ID in order to access the input page, and enter the dosage regimen, plasma concentration-time and initial kinetic values data. After pressing the "Run" button, the data is sent to the Excel® Solver program via the database program and the results are returned within a few seconds in an output page. The output page contains the population, initial and final values of

'V' (volume of distribution) and 'K' (elimination rate constant) along with the observed and predicted plasma concentrations in both tabular and graphic format. Additionally, the user can change "input parameters" and run the program again. Students used this module outside the class to estimate kinetic parameters in simulated scenarios comprising different extents of variability in the plasma concentration and/or the population data. In addition, the module was used during the class time by the teacher for simulation purposes. Not surprisingly, the module significantly improved the student's (outside and inside the class) and teacher's learning of the concepts behind the bayesian forecasting of the kinetic parameters. Further, students felt that the module is easy to use.

3) **Internet-based tutorial to supplement the teaching of medicinal chemistry:** Internet-based tutorial has been developed to supplement the teaching of disease-based medicinal chemistry course. The objectives to develop and implement this tutorial were to: *a*) enhance student's ability to classify and identify drug structures, *b*) provide a chemical rationale supporting the appropriateness of a particular drug or drug class in the treatment of a particular disease or patient, *c*) explain the chemical, biochemical and pharmacological mechanism of drug action and *d*) relate the chemical structure of drugs to their therapeutic actions. The software program ToolBook II Instructor, 5.0 was used to develop the computer tutorial. Web site was designed and created using the Netscape Communicator (version 4.01). The tutorial format found to be significantly different than a simple "computerization" of course lectures. Briefly, adopted tutorial format was such that it revealed vast majority of the course content piece-by-piece through a sequence of questions. The tutorial was subdivided

into four chapters, each of which corresponded to a course lecture sequence. Tutorial page contained a "main index" button which allowed the user to easily move among the four chapters. The designed tutorial consists of hidden questions, 3-D molecular modeling and extended summaries, thereby allowing varying levels of student involvement. A study was conducted to assess student's perceptions of the utility of the tutorials and determine whether students who utilized them fared better on an examination. Based on the student's survey, tutorials were regarded as very useful study aid and adjunct to lecture course material. Two survey instruments were developed and administered at different times during the course. Students conceptualized the utility of the tutorials across two key domains (learning course concepts and developing higher order cognitive skills).

REFERENCES

1. Berge ZL. 2002. Active, interactive, and reflective learning. The Quarterly Review of Distance Education 3:181-190.
2. Carliner S. 1999. Overview of online learning. Amherst MA: Human Resource Development Press.
3. Collison G, Elbaum B, Haavind S, Tinker R. 2000. Facilitating online learning: Effective strategies for moderators. Atwood Publishing, Madison.
4. Greiner A, Knebel E (Eds.). 2003. Health professions education: A bridge to quality. National Academic Press, Washington.
5. Bates T. 1997. The impact of technological change in open and distance learning. Distance Education 18:93-109.
6. Chickering A, Ehrmann S. 1996. Implementing the seven principles: Technology as lever. American Association for Higher Education Bulletin 49:3-6.
7. McGreal R, Elliott M. 2008. Technologies of online learning: E-learning. In T. Anderson (Ed.). Theory and practice of online learning (2nd Ed.). Edmonton, AB: AU Press.
8. Mehvar R. 2000. Development and application of an online module for teaching bayesian forecasting principles in a clinical

pharmacokinetics course. American Journal of Pharmaceutical Education 64:121-125.

9. Harrold MW, Desselle SP. 2000. Development and assessment of an Internet-based tutorial to supplement the teaching of medicinal chemistry within a multidisciplinary, disease-based course. American Journal of Pharmaceutical Education 64:372-380.

10. O'Neil CK, Poirier TI. 2000. Online doctor of pharmacy program for pharmacy practitioners: Development and evaluation of six pilot courses. American Journal of Pharmaceutical Education 64:272-276.

11. Mahoney JS, Marfurt S, DaCunha M, Engebretson J. 2005. Design and evaluation of an online teaching strategy in an undergraduate psychiatric nursing course. Archives of Psychiatric Nursing 19:264-272.

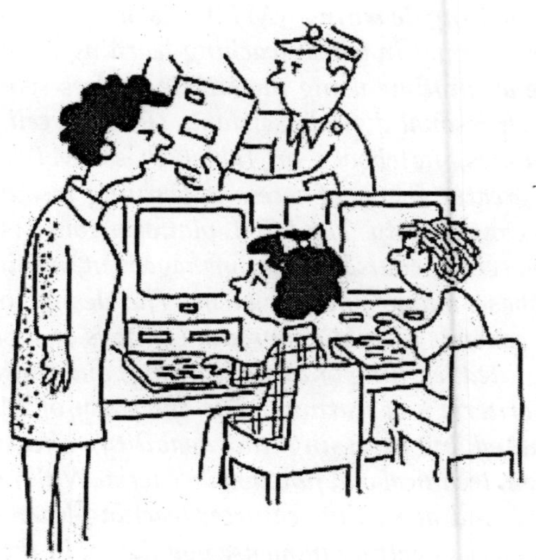

"Emily, have you been shopping online during class."

Chapter 14
MOBILE TEACHING-LEARNING

Kashappa Goud H. Desai

"Whether we like it or not, whether we are ready for it or not, mobile teaching-learning may represent/lead the next innovation in a long tradition of information and communication technologies-based teaching-learning"

Mobile teaching-learning (MT-L) is a very advanced educational format in which teaching-learning is performed anywhere at anytime using the mobile devices (pocket size computers/personal digital assistants (PDAs), cell phones, smart phones, notebooks or Tablet PCs). MT-L format provides greater degree of access to learning resources and powerful connectivity. The MT-L platform consists of MT-L platform server, course content management, result display and database management system. The design of MT-L program consists of study approach (quizzes or assessment or collaborated learning or audio learning) and content, and effective criteria's of learning. The efficiency of MT-L can be evaluated by assessing the usability, effectiveness, satisfaction, technical and functional criteria. With its unique innovative and attractive features, teaching-learning with mobile devices is getting immense popularity in the current technology-based educational system.

INTRODUCTION

From the time of invention of computers, educational technologies have been revolutionizing the ways the teachers teach and the ways the students learn the subjects. The reasons for technological boom in pharmacy education are the potential and attractive advantages that are being offered by the information and communication technologies (ICTs)-based teaching-learning (also known as e-teaching-learning) methods. Unlike traditional teaching, ICTs-based teaching-learning methods provide flexible, interactive, student-centered, collaborative, self-paced, distance and instant learning environment. However, among the numerous ICTs-based teaching-learning methods, Web-based, computer-assisted and online teaching-learning methods received much more attention and acceptance from the educational community. After a successful journey of teaching-learning with ICTs for few decades, there wasn't a feeling of prickly excitement among the educational technologists, faculty and students until another much more attractive educational revolution took place recently. In 2001, introduction of MT-L method brought greater excitement and flexibility for faculty and students/learners, thereby taking the educational status to a new level. Since then, MT-L has become accessible worldwide and receiving immense attraction.

MT-L is the intersection of mobile computing and e-teaching-learning in which teaching-learning process is performed anywhere at anytime utilizing the mobile devices (pocket size computers/personal digital assistants (PDAs), cell phones, smart phones, notebooks or Tablet PCs). Although MT-L is related to the e-teaching-learning and distance education, it is distinct in various aspects of technology, communication and learning context (see Table 14.1).

ADVANTAGES OF MT-L

1) MT-L provides 24/7 access to conventional e-teaching-learning resources and activities.
2) It offers powerful connectivity. This connectivity supports not only contextual access to information, but also synchronous (telephone conversation, voice

Table 14.1

Difference between e-teaching-learning and MT-L programs with respect to technology, modes of communication between teachers and students and methods of evaluation (student's feedback).

No	e-Teaching-Learning	Mobile Teaching-Learning
1.	**Technology**	
	Computer	Mobile devices
	Bandwidth	GPRS, G3, Bluetooth
	Multimedia	Objects
	Interactive	Spontaneous
	Hyperlinked	Connected
	Collaborative	Networked
	Media-rich	Lightweight
	Distance learning	Situated learning
	More formal	Informal
	Simulated situation	Realistic situation
	Hyperlearning	Constructivism, situationism and collaborative
2.	**Modes of communication from teachers to students**	
	Time-delayed (students need to check e-mails or Web sites)	Instant delivery of email or SMS
	Passive communication	Instant communication
	Asynchronous	Synchronous
	Scheduled	Spontaneous
3.	**Modes of communication from students to teachers**	
	Face-to-face	Flexible
	Audio-teleconference common	Audio- and videoconference possible
	e-mail to e-mail	24/7 instantaneous
	Private location	No geographic boundaries
	Travel time to reach Internet site	No travel time since wireless connectivity
	Dedicated time for group meetings	Flexible timings on 24/7 basis
	Poor communication due to group consciousness	Rich communication due to one-to-one communication and reduced inhibitions
4.	**Methods of evaluation**	
	One-to-one basis possible	One-to-one basis possible
	Asynchronous and at times delayed	Both asynchronous and synchronous
	Mass/standardized instruction	Customized instruction
	Benchmark-based grading	Performance & improvement-based grading
	Simulations & lab-based experiments	Real-life cases and on the site experiments
	Paper-based	Less paper, less printing, and lower cost

over Internet protocol (IP), messaging) and asynchronous (Web forums, blog entries, e-mail, text messaging) communication with others.

3) It expands the educational opportunities to undeserved communities in remote areas.
4) It supports locational learning contexts such as field-trips, museums and work-based learning.
5) It enhances interactivity in contact teaching situations
6) It engages 'shy' learners through use of familiar non-threatening technologies (mobile phones).
7) MT-L helps learners to improve their literacy and numeracy skills and recognize their existing abilities.
8) MT-L can be used to encourage both independent and collaborative learning experiences.
9) MT-L helps to remove some of the formality from the learning experience and engages reluctant learners.
10) MT-L helps learners to remain more focused for longer periods.
11) MT-L helps to raise self-esteem and self-confidence.

LIMITATIONS

1) **Infrastructure costs:** MT-L program requires relatively more funding for mobile access devices, developing wireless local area networks (LANs), mobile phone contracts and billing. The important question here is who should provide the mobile devices, institutions or students themselves?

2) **Increased administration and support:** Mobile access devices tend to be less reliable than desktop PCs. Therefore, MT-L takes significant student's training and support for initial set-up, maintenance and troubleshooting mobile access devices.

3) **Managing learning resources:** Microsoft office is used to develop many learning resources. But it is not supported by some mobile access devices. Hence, many Web sites and virtual learning environments are inaccessible to mobile access devices. Therefore, MT-L requires an M-learning portal.

4) **Accessibility:** Mobile phones and PDAs currently have small screens and device controls and can support a limited range of accessibility software.
5) **Increased demands on tutors:** 24/7 access to learning resources may lead to increased demands on tutors.

The above mentioned limitations are listed on the basis of current mobile technological status. These limitations appear to be the future challenges to the educational technologists. Considering the pace at which the educational technology is getting revolutionized, these limitations are likely to be overcome soon by the future technological advancements.

CLASSIFICATION OF MT-L SYSTEM

MT-L system is classified (see below) based on the mobile devices, communication technologies, teacher-student(s) communication, information, access, location and e-teaching-learning standards. This kind of classification provides an opportunity to evaluate the varieties of realizations and requirements to these systems (ICTs (mobile devices and wireless communication technologies) and educational (the type of supported information and the access method to it)).

1) Mobile devices
    a) Notebooks
    b) Tablet PCs
    c) PDAs
    d) Cell phones
    e) Smart phones
2) Wireless communication technologies
    a) General packet radio service (GPRS)
    b) Global system for mobile communications (GSM)
    c) IEEE 802.11
    d) Bluetooth
    e) Infrared data association (IrDA)

3) Communication between teachers and students
    a) Synchronous
    b) Asynchronous
4) Information
    a) Learning materials
    b) Administrative information
5) Access
    a) On-line
    b) Off-line
6) Location
    a) On-campus
    b) Off-campus
7) e-teaching-learning standards
    a) Supported
    b) Non-supported

MOBILE TEACHING-LEARNING PLATFORM

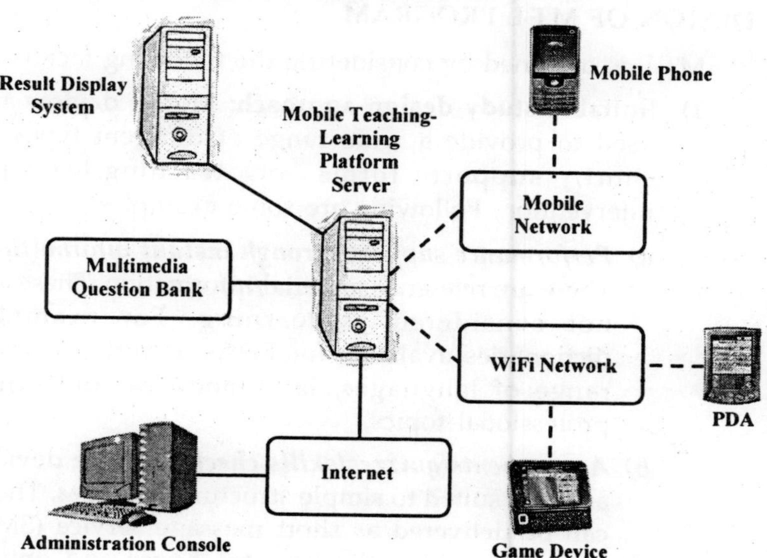

Figure 14.1. Mobile teaching-learning platform

The mobile teaching-learning platform generally consists of a mobile teaching-learning server, course content management system, result display system and database management system (see Figure 14.1). Through the campus-wide wireless fidelity (WiFi) network, students can use mobile devices including PDA, mobile phones or mobile gaming devices to log-in to the mobile learning platform and then test their own knowledge anytime and anywhere. In addition, this mobile teaching-learning platform can aid each course teacher to closely monitor the learning pace or progress of each individual student/group. The display system can spontaneously display the student's answer and his/her attained grade/mark in a real-time manner, thus allowing the teacher to correct the student's common mistakes on the spot. Furthermore, the teacher will be informed of the student's learning pace through this real-time report system to quickly adjust the teaching progress or materials.

DESIGN OF MT-L PROGRAM

MT-L is designed by considering the following factors.

1) **Suitable study design approach:** Mobile devices are used to provide a wide range of different types of short, support forms of teaching-learning intervention. Following are some examples.

   a) ***Performance support through instant information:*** These are reference material/information. These are not considered as learning. For example, dictionaries available for PDAs, covering a wide range of languages, law, medicine and other professional topics.

   b) ***Assessments/quizzes/skills checks:*** Mobile devices are well suited to simple structured quizzes. These can be delivered as short message service (SMS) messages asking the user to choose and option and respond, possibly with a deadline. Feedback from a teacher (as a SMS message) is also an example.

c) ***Collaborative learning***: Examples are SMS/voice/e-mail contact with a teacher (if part of a blended programme with teacher support), participation in polls via SMS, instant messaging facilities (available on many smart phones), and sharing of information via uploads to a central location (using multimedia messaging service (MMS) functionality).

d) ***Audio learning***: The devices used are iPod, MP3 and mobile phones. Examples include site-specific inductions, interviews, course offerings and revision aids.

e) ***Video learning***: Mobile devices are used to play video clips for teaching-learning

2) Suitable study content: After considering and deciding about study design approach, educators need to decide about the specific content types for mobile teaching-learning process.

a) Simple and self-contained processes, where specific knowledge should be retrieved/accessed in a certain moment.

b) Topics where ability to locate in a specific time/place adds value.

c) Topics where best practice and advice tips can be easily packaged and presented.

d) Topics where expert opinions and viewpoints can add value (through audio and/or video).

e) Topics where the target audience is more likely to benefit from access to learning on the move

3) Criteria's for effective teaching-learning design

a) Keep it short

b) Keep it simple

c) Apply a structure
d) Use media judiciously
e) Make access easy
f) Provide opportunities for collaboration

MT-L PROGRAM IN MAINSTREAM EDUCATION: INCLUSION CRITERIA

There are four essential criteria that should be considered while including the MT-L program in mainstream education. These include: enrolment of mobile learning students on the institution's official prospectus and into fee-paying, assessed and accredited courses. If these processes are not done, MT-L remains peripheral and may not be considered as part of mainstream provision.

EVALUATION OF MT-L PROGRAM

The evaluation of MT-L program can be performed based on the need of the evaluators (what the evaluators want to know). Therefore, based on the objective of the evaluation, one or all of the criteria given below can be used.

1) **Usability:** This criterion is concerned to the easiness of understanding, learning, remembering and using the device and its tools. Following are the key device and tools usability criteria that need to be evaluated.

    a) User-interface: User-interface parameters include: 1) appropriate and effective layout, 2) simple and easy to use menu, toolbars, buttons etc, 3) multiple languages, 4) personalization and various versions and 5) accommodation and special needs person's consideration.

    ***b) Presentation and media*:** These include: 1) easy to read, write, draw, record (photo, audio, video etc.), play and print, 2) variety of media support (text, diagrams, maps, photos, sound, video etc.) and 3) quality and fidelity of multimedia.

c) ***Navigation***: The parameters include: *1*) simple and easy structure/organization, *2*) effective and easy organization of files, *3*) effective and easy organization of tools and functions, *4*) simple and easy navigation, *5*) shortcuts available, *6*) return to home from everywhere, *7*) help from everywhere, *8*) search from everywhere, *9*) no broken and missing links, *10*) simple and consistent orientation everywhere, *11*) table of contents, *12*) directories for email addresses, telephone numbers, radio stations, TV stations, etc, and *13*) directories for emails, SMS, MMS, calls, files, photos, songs, etc.

2) **Effectiveness:** The effectiveness of mobile MT-L program depends on the educational aims and context. Thus, any assessment of the effects of MT-L program must be related to the context of the activity and its intended aims. The important questions that the evaluators need to ask themselves are: *a*) is the aim to learn a topic or to develop specific skills or to support incidental and lifelong learning? and *b*) is it initiated and managed by the learner or externally?

3) **Satisfaction:** Satisfaction with mobile learning is superficially the easiest to assess, through attitude surveys (use of questionnaire comprising questions about the program satisfaction) or interviews with students/learners.

4) **Technical:** In this criterion, device's performance, connectivity, compatibility, security and reliability parameters are to be evaluated. These include: *1*) the device should have high processing power, large available memory and ability to run various software formats, *2*) the device should have long battery autonomy and easy battery recharging, *3*) the device should support various communication protocols and networks without serious restrictions on distance and bandwidth and *4*) the device should also secure

the content and communications against theft or malicious changes.

5) **Functional:** This criterion is related to the quantity and quality of the available features, functions and tools of the device. It should support tools for synchronous and asynchronous communication and information access, processing, storage, organization and playing.

Barriers in Evaluating the MT-L Program

Evaluating the MT-L program is a very difficult and challenging task for the educators. The barriers of evaluation are associated with the advantages being provided by the MT-L method. Following are key barriers associated with the evaluation of MT-L program.

1) ***MT-L may be mobile (but not necessarily)***: If the learner is travelling while learning, it is not easy to capture as there may be no fixed point in time or space to locate an observer or a video camera. It becomes further difficult when learning involves multiple participants and distributed over many locations.

2) ***MT-L may occur in non-formal settings***: Many studies of mobile learning may occur in non-formal educational settings (e.g., museums and field trips).

3) ***MT-L may be extended and interleaved***: An appealing aspect of MT-L is that it can support the learner over a long period of time. Therefore, it is not be possible to determine when the learning begins and ends, nor when a person is deliberately learning or just enjoying an activity (which itself may lead to unintended learning).

4) ***MT-L may involve a variety of personal and institutional technologies***: Sometimes, students move around the campus to use other institutional technologies (set-up). Therefore, it is very difficult to

evaluate numerous technologies for one educational program.

5) ***MT-L presents particular ethical problems***: These include getting permission from all participants to be monitored for research purposes and allowing participants the right to choose when to be monitored.

MOBILE TECHNOLOGIES IN PHARMACY EDUCATION/PRACTICE

In the health care system, pharmacy practitioners play crucial role by providing information on medications-related issues. Currently, pharmacists provide medications-related information in person or through computer network/e-mail. Mobile technologies (mobile access) can provide greater flexibility for pharmacists to work promptly and efficiently. These technologies can give mobile access to key health care information which in turn improves patient's outcomes and satisfy physicians with prompt support. In particular, these technologies give access to real-time patient's information and clinical references and retrieve real-time patient's data on rounds. With portable mobile devices (e.g., mobile phone or PDA), detailed drug information, latest patient records and laboratory values will be at their fingertips. Further, pharmacists with wireless tablet personal computers or PDAs can readily answer the medications-related questions and speed-up the patient's treatments. Based on the service of pharmacists, appropriate software can be loaded onto the mobile devices (for example, drug information software) and used to provide the required service. Some of the software include: *a*) MedCalc/MedMath medical equation software, *b*) Lexi-CALC (which calculates infusions and converts pediatric and adult doses), *c*) Lexi-Comp drug information with FDA alerts, *d*) APK (a pharmacokinetic dosing program), and *e*) Clinical Xpert CareFocus (a Web- and mobile-based patient-profiling system that is part of Thomson Healthcare's Mercury MD and can define alert situations among high-risk patients).

REFERENCES

1. Corlett D, Sharples M, Chan T, Bull S. 2004. A mobile learning organizer for university students. Paper presented at the 2nd International workshop on wireless and mobile technologies in education, JungLi, Taiwan.
2. Davis S. 2003. Observations in classrooms using a network of handheld devices. Journal of Computer Assisted Learning 19:298-307.
3. Dawabi P, Wessner M, Neuhold E. 2003. Using mobile devices for the classroom of the future. Paper presented at the M-learn 2003 on learning with mobile devices, London.
4. Houser C, Thornton P, Kluge D. 2002. Mobile learning: Cell phones and PDAs for education. Paper presented at the International conference on computers in education, Auckland, New Zealand.
5. Patten B, Sanchez AI, Tangney B. 2006. Designing collaborative, constructionist and contextual applications for handheld devices. Computers and Education 46:294-308.
6. Smørdal O, Gregory J. 2003. Personal digital assistants in medical education and practice. Journal of Computer Assisted Learning 19:320-329.

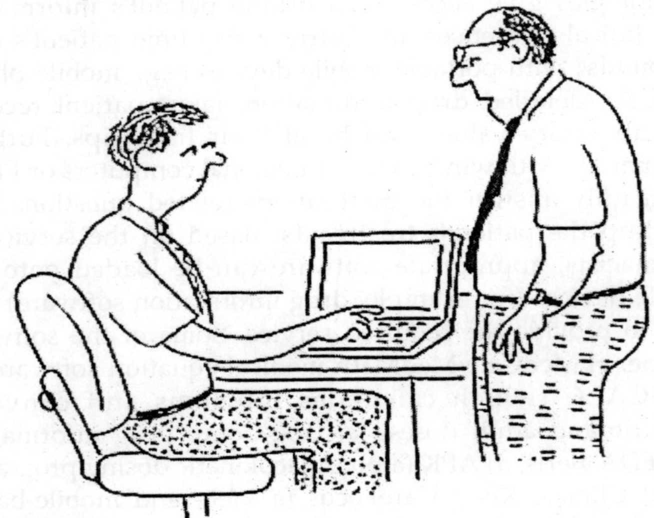

"When I was a student, wireless data transmission meant passing notes in class."

Chapter 15
PHARMACY INFORMATICS

Shobha Churi

When a thing was new, people said, "It is not true". When the truth became obvious, people said, "It is not important". When its importance could not be denied, people said, "Any way, it is not new"

—William James

Pharmacy informatics is an interface where the computers and appropriate technologies are used to store, retrieve, analyze, use and disseminate the drug and prescription information. A four-layer (foundation, management information, decision support and advanced information system layer) hierarchy of information systems is utilized in health care system. If the medical professionals become experts in the health informatics (automation in the process of generation and reviewing medication order and examining relevant variables and suggesting the alternatives), the role of pharmacists in health care system will be in jeopardy. Since the current pharmacy curriculum does not include the complete use of advanced informatics, pharmacy educational institutions need to take the responsibility to implement advanced informatics in the curriculum and practice of pharmacy. Teaching today with advanced informatics is a step towards preparing the students for tomorrow's challenge (pharmacy informaticists). Pharmacy informaticists will then need to monitor its subsequent application and use it to enhance their worth on the health care team and improve patient care.

INTRODUCTION

The introduction of first generation pharmacy-specific computer technology in the field of pharmacy practice, particularly for retail and hospital pharmacy services, took place in 1970s through 1990s. The term pharmacy informatics is much newer than the domain it specifies. Recently, with the introduction of advanced information technology, the trend in pharmacy informatics has moved from pharmacy-specific system to larger, fully-integrated information system that include pharmacy functions as a component of larger clinical information, retail prescription management and drug supply chain management system. In addition, computerized provider order entry for medication orders in hospitals and electronic prescribing (e-Prescribing) of prescriptions (sent via networks from physician offices to retail pharmacies) has also been introduced. More recently, there has been significant development in pharmacy informatics professional activity. Hospitals and their pharmacy departments are adding more medication-related software applications, automated storage and distribution devices, electronic infusion devices, electronic medication administration records, bar-coding technology and electronic medical and health record systems at an accelerated pace. These activities have resulted in unprecedented collaborations to improve the safety, quality and productivity of medication-use systems, but much remains to be done to ensure widespread and effective dissemination of these technologies.

Pharmacy informatics, a subset of pharmacoinformatics (discipline where technology intersects with any aspect of drug delivery, from the basic sciences (e.g. drug development or pharmacogenomics/pharmacogenetics) to the clinical use of medications in individuals and populations), typically refers to the interface of information technology with the practice of pharmacy. In other words, pharmacy informatics is an interface where the computers and appropriate technologies are used to store, retrieve, analyze, use and disseminate the drug and prescription information.

Why 'Advanced Informatics' is Necessary in the Curriculum and Practice of Pharmacy?

There are numerous reasons why 'informatics' is necessary in the curriculum and practice of pharmacy. Informatics is the use of information technology to enhance the quality of patient care, facilitate accountability and assist in cost containment. The information backbone or information infrastructure used by the health system is critical to pharmacy's mission. Without the integrated informatics system, it is difficult to provide high-quality patient care and contain the costs. Unlike the allied medical professionals, pharmacists have a slight lead in decision-support system. Therefore, pharmacists can use 'informatics' to promote their involvement in the health care system. Importantly, other disciplines are making decisions about information system design that could create roles for non-pharmacists. The roles of non-pharmacists can be best filled by the pharmacists. Hence, implementation of advanced informatics in the curriculum and practice of pharmacy is highly essential. Pharmacists will need to monitor its application and use it to enhance their worth on the health care team and improve patient care.

ROLES OF PHARMACY INFORMATICS

1) Act as computerized prescriber order entry, electronic health records and clinical decision-support system.
2) A system to generate clear, useful and accurate medication administration records.
3) A system to generate drug usage evaluation reports.
4) Tool to place purchase orders.
5) Inventory tracking system.
6) Act as a system for accessing clinical information such as laboratory reports and drug interaction details.
7) Potential medium to educate patients/staff/students.
8) Assist in qualitative and quantitative research (act as instantly available information system for

searching thousands of patient records for adverse drug events with great efficiency).

9) Assists and enables experimental and clinical studies to be conducted in an entirely different and more efficient manner.

10) Management tool for bar-coded medications.

INFORMATION HIERARCHY IN THE PRACTICE OF PHARMACY

A four-layer hierarchy of information system is utilized in health care system. Understanding the current status of information system helps to determine how the advanced informatics functions.

1) **Layer 1:** It is a foundation layer of computer-based information which is formed by a transaction-processing system. For example, medication order processing.

2) **Layer 2:** This layer is the management information system (MIS). In this layer, computer generates reports that give feedback to managers on what trends are occurring in the transaction layer below. For example, drug-use reports and inventory management reports.

3) **Layer 3:** The third layer is decision support system. A good decision-support system provides instantaneous access to information in a just-in-time manner. For example, drug-use review screening database. Most pharmacy management systems flag potential drug-related problems. Additionally, some pharmacy management systems assist in suggesting the alternatives and helps with final decision-making.

4) **Layer 4:** The fourth layer is information system comprising advanced informatics applications. Health care system is increasingly using this advanced system to support patient care. These applications include the use of expert systems, artificial intelligence, fuzzy logic and neural networks.

THE NEED FOR STANDARDS

A barrier to informatics progress is the lack of information standards in the industry. Today, the typical health care system runs a conglomeration of information applications. Many of these offer no compatibility for data exchange with other systems. The lack of data exchange standards forces an additional layer of expense, in the form of interfacing technology required for the existing system. Thus, there is a need to develop industry-wide standards of communication for the health care field. Standards make it easier for stand-alone applications to communicate. Provision for exchange of information from different software applications leads to successful implementation of pharmacy informatics.

THE FUTURE OF PHARMACY INFORMATICS

If appropriate standards are set and vendors cooperate, more and more advanced informatics applications will talk to one another. As a result, different systems within the same department will share information more easily. This will happen at all levels: between departments and between institutions. Further, health care processes will be integrated, personnel will be used more effectively, costs will be contained and the right information will reach the right people when they need it, thereby improving the patient's health care. The G7 leaders are supporting the 'global healthcare applications project' as an effort to shape the future of health care. In fact, eleven projects are underway to share databases and technology to improve, present, prevent, diagnose and treat diseases, aid in disease surveillance and assist in research.

In the future, experts may develop patient-specific formulary. This formulary will not be a smashed-down group of drugs from which providers will select. Instead, it will be that subset of all drugs that produce a desired therapeutic effect in an individual patient (and population).

In the advanced health care system, the physician will perform the health care processes (generation and reviewing of medication order by using the personal digital assistant and prospective drug-use review module, respectively and examining relevant variables and suggesting the alternatives by using an expert system) utilizing the health informatics. Where is the pharmacist? In this scenario, pharmacists may not be in the loop. Hence, some pharmacists fear that advanced health care informatics will be the death of the role of pharmacists. However, in certain cases, pharmacy informaticists become necessary. For example, in case if the decision is not 'clean' but requires information that is missing or that has an unacceptable confidence level, pharmacy informaticists are necessary to make the medication-related decisions.

PREPARING FUTURE PHARMACY INFORMATICISTS

Pharmacy educational institutions must respond to constantly growing informatics. Informatics needs to be included as a course and keep alive as a common denominator in the pharmacy course. While applying informatics internally to the pharmacy department, automation of information flow for processes that already exist is not advisable. Informatics should be approached in the beginning by determining where the department is going strategically. Once that is known, enabling steps should be then taken by the pharmacy students. It is advisable that department starts with the basics and the literature will give clues about practical innovations.

Unfortunately, Indian pharmacy students are not receiving in-depth exposure to the principles and practice of advanced pharmacy informatics. Note that some US pharmacy colleges have already included pharmacy informatics in their curriculum and training the students to prepare them for the future challenge. Pharmacy educators in India must respond to the initiatives across the globe and evolving technology within the profession. In other words, they have to embrace the term pharmacy informatics and develop a standardized pharmacy informatics curriculum.

Within pharmacy education, informatics can be defined as the science that uses digital information to improve pharmaceutical outcomes and student learning. Given below are strategies to embed the pharmacy informatics in the curriculum.

Implementing 'Pharmacy Informatics' in the Pharmacy Practice/PharmD Curriculum

The systematic implementation of 'pharmacy informatics' in the pharmacy practice or PharmD curriculum involves five central domains. The tasks to be done in each domain are discussed below.

1) ***Domain one: Student exit (future) competencies in informatics***: This domain guides colleges and curriculum planners in developing focused topical content in informatics and related automated systems/technology within the pharmacy practice/PharmD curriculum. 'Expertise' (knowledge of informatics and the application of existing and emerging technologies into practice) in informatics has been identified as one of the required competencies for students.

    a) Development of foundational training within colleges of pharmacy is required. The learning topics in this training segment should range from basic computer science knowledge (data management, warehousing, electronic communications between people or systems and architecture of systems) to applications (automation, smart systems, decision support, computers in patient safety, medical coding, information reliability, retrieval and literacy).

    b) Educators should collaborate to develop acceptable discipline-wide standards and guidelines on educational outcomes.

    c) Each college should periodically define its own student's performance, exit competencies and best practices with corresponding curricular mapping in the informatics/technology realm.

d) While developing the curriculum, planning committee should give consideration to basic evaluative skill sets and needs analysis in: *1*) the accuracy and authority of professional, scientific and online information, 2) electronic documentation skills from the first week of the curriculum to the last day of the advanced pharmacy practice experience, *3*) use of the electronic medical record as well as recognizing the significance of the availability to specific patient information from any practice setting, *4*) review of current healthcare informatics in the marketplace and *5*) informing students of data security and confidentiality issues.

e) The curriculum should also include 'teaching of clinical decision support systems'. With this segment, students gain knowledge and skills in evaluating available software, will know about effective and efficient use of software/appliance within a patient-centered systems practice approach, and will be capable of adapting their knowledge and practices to smart systems, future applications and innovations.

2) ***Domain two: Informatics as an aid to students learning***: The objective to embed the technology in teaching and teaching about technology is to inculcate in students an appreciation for the critical importance of technology. To achieve this objective, curriculum must include not only the integration of informatics but also the use of other technology-based teaching-learning methods (computer-assisted and Web-based teaching-learning, interactive learning, multimedia, multi-user and discussion board formats). Collaboration among colleges to gather the necessary resources are vital in achieving this goal. Tutorials and interactive simulation laboratories are considered as effective educational teaching-learning methods. Interactive simulation laboratories include the potential for the development of teaching tools such as cyber-patients, cyber-rounds and cyber-cases for consistent, stimulating and accessible student learning and assessment.

3) ***Domain three*: *Support for individual faculty efforts in promoting informatics*:** Pharmacy educators and administrators need to work together to achieve successful implementation of pharmacy informatics in the curriculum. While doing so, the primary hurdles are likely to appear in the areas of skills, costs and recognition. Administrators need to develop a culture that empowers pharmacy educators in the area of informatics. For example, include informatics and educational technology as areas for routine faculty development. Educational costs are a constant concern for administration, but sufficient financial resources must be made available for informatics to be successfully implemented within college curricula. Administrators need to find ways to facilitate the expansion of informatics within pharmacy curricula and provide recognition (promotion, incentives etc.) to those educators who commit significant time and effort to this task.

4) ***Domain four: Academic leadership within healthcare pharmacy informatics*:** Outside of the informatics domain, pharmacist is considered as a drug use and monitoring experts. Due to the nature of ubiquitous user-friendly drug information software, the traditional drug expert resource role of pharmacists is under risk. Therefore, tomorrow's pharmacists should become the leaders in the use of robotic and distributive systems throughout the healthcare

Table 15.1
Student's evaluation questionnaire for pharmacy informatics (PI) course[a]

	Question/Statement	% Response				
		5	4	3	2	1
1	Already exposed to PI before					
2	Knowledge of PI was sufficient before this course					
3	Course content not sufficient and/or not comprehensive					
4	Course not well conducted					
5	Knowledge about PI increased after the course					
6	Course was too imaginative					
7	Course was up-to-date					
8	Course should be marinated					
9	I learned about use of Internet/network in patient's health care					
10	Coursework was appropriate					
11	Coursework was interesting and stimulating					
12	Course was not related to lecture contents					
13	Assistance and guidance not given during coursework					
14	Facilities other than computers are sufficient					
15	Computers available not enough					
16	Time allocated for the coursework was sufficient					

Likert scale: 1= Strongly Disagree; 2= Disagree; 3= Neutral; 4= Agree; 5= Strongly Agree.
[a] Based on Rahman et al.

enterprise. To become an expert/leader, pharmacist should be allowed to involve in software design and development. Among the new, often inexperienced (untried) and frequently conflicting sources of drug information, the role of pharmacist as the authoritative voice should be maintained. Therefore, tomorrow's pharmacist should be more knowledgeable, skillful and responsive than ever before to maintain a viable and leading role in the advanced healthcare process.

5) ***Domain five: Graduate programs in pharmacy informatics***: In the constantly evolving and challenging profession of pharmacy practice, the future necessity (pharmacy academic leadership in healthcare informatics) demand the graduate programs in various aspects of informatics. Therefore, administrators/curriculum planners need to develop numerous course/programs for the students (residency, graduate, PharmD, doctoral degree etc). Further, collaborative efforts should be undertaken to provide education and training opportunities in informatics for faculty members.

Evaluation of Pharmacy Informatics Course/Program

Student's questionnaires can be used to evaluate the pharmacy informatics course. The questions can be designed based on a five-point Likert scale (see Table 15.1). Open-ended questions will provide student's opinions and comments about the course. Students should be allowed to provide strengths and weakness of the course. Getting student's suggestions to improve/modify the course framework can also be part of evaluation.

REFERENCES

1. Flynn AJ. 2005. Implementing pharmacy informatics in college curricula: The AACP technology in pharmacy education and learning special interest group. American Journal of Pharmaceutical Education 69:490-494.

2. Clark T. 2007. Adopting health care informatics and technologies. American Journal of Health-System Pharmacy 64:145.

3. Hope C. 2007. Influence of pharmacy informatics on research. American Journal of Health-System Pharmacy 64:237.
4. Siska MH, Meyer GE. 2008. Pharmacy informatics: Aligning for success. American Journal of Health-System Pharmacy 65:1410-1411.
5. Ball MJ, Douglas JV. 1990. Informatics programs in the United States and abroad. M D Computing 7:172-175.
6. Barker KN, Allan EL, Swensson ES. 1989. Effect of technological changes in information transfer on the delivery of pharmacy services. American Journal of Pharmaceutical Education 53:27-40.
7. Ball MJ, Douglas JV, Zimmerman JL. 1989. Informatics education and the professions. Journal of the American Society for Information Science 40:368-377.
8. Scott MG, McElnay JC, Burnett KM. 1996. Using bar-code technology to capture clinical intervention data in a hospital with a stand-alone pharmacy computer system. American Journal of Health-System Pharmacy 53:651-4.
9. Felkey B. 1995. The role of medical informatics and automation in future health care systems. International Pharmacy Journal 9:108-110.
10. Rahman AFA, Ibrahim MIM, Bahari MB, Mohamed MHN. 2002. Design and evaluation of the pharmacoinformatics course at pharmacy school in Malaysia. Drug Information Journal 36:783-789.

Chapter 16

TRADITIONAL AND MODERN TEACHING-LEARNING MEDIA/AIDS

Shobha Churi

Teaching-learning media/aids are used as tools by teachers to help students improve reading and other skills, illustrate or reinforce a skill, fact and idea, and relieve anxiety, fears and boredom. These aids stimulate, motivate and capture student's attention, thereby reinforcing the learning process. Teaching-learning media/aids help teachers to impart educational information to the students effectively. These range from written/printed materials to audiovisual equipment to eChalk system. Depending on the mode of teaching-learning, appropriate medium is used.

INTRODUCTION

The educational process is conducted with a proper educational objective. To achieve the educational objectives, teacher use suitable teaching-learning method and medium. Role of a teacher is to impart and emphasize information effectively to the students. From the time the traditional teaching method has introduced, oral communication has been a popular teaching-learning medium. However, oral communication alone offers some limitations. For example, in listening, only 20% of what is heard is remembered, whereas in visual more than 40% of what is seen is retained in memory. The retention in memory is more than 70% if seen and heard. Introduction of variety of other media/aids have led to significant improvement in the quality of teaching-learning. Teaching-learning media/aids stimulate, motivate and capture student's attention, thereby reinforcing the learning process. Such media/aids are actually components of teaching-learning methods. Variety of teaching-learning media/aids are used in teaching/learning process which range from simple (written/printed materials) to sophisticated (eChalk system). Depending on the mode of teaching/learning, appropriate teaching-learning medium/aid can be used. Following are the commonly used and modern teaching-learning media/aids.

TYPES OF TEACHING-LEARNING MEDIA/AIDS

As the teaching-learning methods are getting revolutionized with time, newer and attractive teaching-learning media/aids are being introduced. Following are the traditional and modern teaching-learning media/aids. Based on the teaching-learning method, audience size (small or large group) and advantages and disadvantages associated with the media/aids, suitable medium/aid should be selected for teaching-learning process. Due to potential benefits (highly attractive, inevitable in teaching-learning complex topics, highly flexible, convenient to use and speedy use) of the advanced teaching-learning media/aids, many of the traditional media/aids have become obsolete. Therefore, in the forthcoming sections, more widely used and modern media/aids are discussed in detail.

1) Visual aids
   - A) Non-projected visual aids
     - a) Chalk board
     - b) White board
     - c) Flip charts
   - B) Projected visual aids
     - a) Overhead projector (OHP) and transparency sheets
     - b) Liquid crystal display (LCD) projector

c) eChalk-system

d) Slide projector, episcope, microprojector and direct projector

2) Audio aids

A) Public address system

B) Audiotape system/audio compact disc (CD)

3) Audio visual aids

A) Videotape system/films

B) Virtual reality

4) Written aids

5) Patients and real objects

6) Three dimensional representations

A) Models

B) Simulators

7) Role play

8) Mass communication

A) Radio

B) Television

1) **Visual aids:** Visual media/aids are powerful tools for effective communication. These media/aids increase the understanding, save time, enhance retention and promote attentiveness. Visual aids range from simple handled objects to multi-media. Based on the size of the audience, information to be conveyed, physical environment of the room, equipment available, time available to prepare visual aids, affordability and advantages and disadvantages associated with visual aid, suitable aid/medium should be selected for the teaching-learning process. Following are the sub-types of visual aids.

A) Non-projected visual aids

a) Chalk board: It is a conventional aid and has been using from several decades. Chalk board is available in black and green color. In spite of availability of advanced teaching-learning media/ aids, the conventional chalk board is still unsurpassed as teaching medium. This is mainly because of its simplicity, intuitive use and unmatched flexibility. It is useful for teaching the group of 30-50 students.

Advantages

1) Economical (initial investment and maintenance is minimal).
2) Easily accessible in most of the lecture rooms.
3) Working on chalk board supports creative thinking, illustration and sharing.
4) Supports in following the conceptual process.
5) Material written on the board can be retained for a longer duration which enables students to take notes during the session.
6) Easy and flexible to use.
7) Electricity and technical devices are not required for its use.
8) No need of darkening the room.

Disadvantages

1) Eye-to-eye contact is lost with students while writing.
2) Material written on the board cannot be stored and reused for future.
3) Preparation of material in advance is not possible.
4) Requires certain drawing and writing skills from the teacher.
5) Drawing diagrams consumes lots of time and space.
6) Teachers and students may be allergic to chalk dust.

Tips for use

Do's

1) Start the lecture with clean board.
2) Write only key points.
3) Write the lecture contents in step-by-step concept.
4) Write large and clear letters by applying sufficient pressure.
5) Use white or yellow colored chalk for writing the contents. For highlighting the other contents or drawing the diagrams, use different colored chalks.
6) Use the area of the board systematically by dividing into three equal parts and using in the order.
7) Erase the board contents in order in which it is written.
8) At the end of the lecture, wipe the board cleanly.

Don'ts

1) Don't write at the corners and bottom of the board. Because the sentences may not be visible to the students sitting in the last row.
2) Don't talk while writing on the board.

b) White board: White board is the modern teaching medium. It has smooth and shiny surface on which teachers can write easily and wipe cleanly. White board requires several color pens which are specially designed for white board teaching. The white boards are available in various dimensions. Small portable white boards are also used as flip charts. Compared to the black board, the additional advantages of white board are: *1*) there is no problem of dust allergy and 2) highly flexible (board height can be adjusted). The disadvantage of white board over the black board is that it is relatively expensive.

Tips to use

Do's

1) Start the lecture with clean board.
2) Write large and clear letters.
3) Use erasable white board pens.
4) Use the area of the board systematically by dividing into three equal parts and using them in the order.
5) Write only key points and develop conceptual structure of the lecture.
6) After use, cover the pens with cap to get long durability.
7) At the end of the lecture, clean the board properly.

Don'ts

1) Don't use permanent marker.
2) Don't write at the corner and bottom of the board.
3) Don't talk while writing on the board.

c) *Flip charts*: Flip charts are inexpensive and can be prepared quickly. Flip charts are suitable for briefing a small group. These help the speaker to proceed through the material and convey information efficiently. These can be prepared prior to as well as during the presentation. Further, these can be used to document audience questions and comments. The raw materials (paper, color pens and stand) are easily available and less expensive.

Advantages

1) Can be prepared prior to presentation.
2) Can be used to write the feedback and comment of the students.
3) Easy to handle.

4) Doesn't require great expertise for preparation.
5) Can be used to highlight and summarize the points during the session.

Disadvantages

1) May require the graphical talent.
2) Not suitable for teaching the large group.
3) Difficult to transport.
4) Unreadable handwriting is disadvantage, but can be overcome by printed material.

Tips to prepare

Do's

1) Each sheet of paper should contain one idea or sketch or theme.
2) The size of words, charts and diagrams should be large enough to be seen by the students clearly.
3) Use block letters and size of the letters should be at least 5 cm.
4) Use capital letters and don't slant or italicize the letters.
5) Use different colored pens to make it more attractive and effective.
6) Show only the key points of the lecture.

Don'ts

1) Don't write the lecture contents at the bottom of the flip chart as it is not visible to the students sitting in the back row.
2) Don't write the whole lecture contents on the paper.

B) *Projected visual aids*

a) OHP and transparency sheets: The transparency sheets are used to write the lecture contents and

OHP is used to project the transparency sheet's contents on a screen or wall. OHP and transparency sheets are useful aid for teaching a group of 20 to 50 studer ts. Teaching with this aid (OHP and transparency sheets) maintains eye-to-eye contact with students and do not consume too much time to prepare the transparencies. Hence, this is a powerful teaching aid. The lecture contents can be written on the sheets with the marker pens (special pens made for writing on the transparency sheets) or photocopied onto the sheets. For writing the contents, thinner transparency sheets (50-75 microns) can be used. Two types of pens (water soluble and water indelible) can be used for writing. Water soluble ink can be easily removed by washing or using wet cloth. Water indelible ink is removed by alcohol. Whereas, for photocopying the lecture contents onto the sheets, relatively thicker transparency sheets (100 microns) are required. OHP is a device used to project the OHP sheet's contents onto a screen or wall. The OHP consists of a bright lamp, lens system and mirror. For a better clarity projection, projector and screen should be adjusted and arranged precisely. Place the projector on a relatively smaller table than the surrounding tables or platform to make it less imposing. The screen should be completely visible to all students and placed above the level of speaker's head. The location of OHP and screen should be such that arrangement should provide the least obstructed view (45-degree angle to the students).

Advantages

1) No need to darken the room.
2) Eye-to-eye contact is not lost.

3) Material (transparencies) can be prepared in advance and can be reused in future.
4) Easy to carry the transparencies.
5) Handling of projector is simple.

Disadvantages

1) Electricity is essential, alternate arrangements should be made in case of power failure.
2) Some speakers feel captive to the machine as they must change each transparency sheet by hand.
3) Sometimes, the projected image size is too small to be seen by the students sitting in the last row of a large room.
4) It is difficult to write on the transparency sheet while it is on the projector.

Tips to prepare transparency sheets

Do's

1) Write the lecture contents as 'points' rather than sentences.
2) The letters should be clear and at least 8 mm in height. Uniformity in style and size of the letters should be maintained.
3) If possible, use stencil or templates for hand writing.
4) Use different colored markers to prepare a sheet. It captures the student's attention and differentiates the lecture concepts.
5) Restrict less than 8 words per line and 6 lines per sheet.
6) Photocopying the lecture contents onto transparency sheets is much better option than writing. It gives better clarity. However, it is hard to differentiate the lecture contents.

Don'ts

1) Don't talk while looking at the screen, talk by looking at the students.
2) Don't unveil the full sheet at once. Cover the sheet with the paper and disclose the points one-by-one.

b) *Liquid crystal display (LCD) projector*: LCD projector is simple, smaller and more portable projection device. LCD projector consists of metal halide lamps. These lamps can project an image on any flat surface. To use this projection device, one should first prepare the presentation slides using the computer and appropriate software (Microsoft® PowerPoint and supportive software). Then, by connecting the LCD projector and computer, prepared slides can be projected on the screen or wall. Material from floppy/CD/pen drive can also be projected using the computer. In recent time, it has become a widely used visual aid in education. Using the appropriate screen (small or large), this aid can be used for small and large group teaching.

Advantages

1) Professional in appearance.
2) Slides can be prepared in advance.
3) Easy to carry the slides.
4) Easy to integrate with classroom discussion.
5) Easy to update and revise the slides contents.
6) Video clippings can be incorporated into the presentation/slides to make the students understand the subject clearly.

Disadvantages

1) Initial investment is high (LCD projector is very expensive).

2) Require computer knowledge and initial training to use.
3) Require significant time to prepare high quality slides.
4) Uninterrupted electricity is necessary.

Tips to prepare slides

Do's

1) Keep the objective for the presentation (what you want to convey).
2) Font style and font size: For main title, use Arial or San Serif font style. San Serif is easier to read. Avoid italics. Font size needs to be between 28-48 points. Use bold and regular font.
3) Other contents: Font size needs to be between 24-30 points. Use Arial or San Serif font style. Use normal and bold letters.
4) Write six words per sentence and six line/points per slide.
5) Use key phrases as far as possible.
6) Maintain logical flow from beginning to end.
7) Use clearly visible color combination.
8) Use bullets or numbers for writing each point.
9) Projection screen should be of good clarity.
10) Carry the material in more than one device (e.g., floppy, CD, and pen drive).
11) If necessary, load the presentation materials into the designated computer in advance.
12) Before transferring the presentation materials to the designated computer, check the configuration and compatibility of the computer you used to prepare slides with that of one you use for presentation.
13) Prepare presentation handout. The concept/points to be covered in each slide should be written in a handout.

Don'ts

1) Don't overload the slides with lots of concepts or results or data. Use only the contents, results and data necessary for fulfilling the objective of the presentation. Remaining contents, results and data can be placed in the supportive presentation slides.
2) Don't use too many animations to present the slides. Audience becomes impatient or loose interest with too many animations.

c) *eChalk system:* Inspired by the features of chalkboard, electronic chalk (eChalk) system has been developed. eChalk system (software) is a very modern teaching-learning aid which consists of a pen-based input device and wide display. In addition to writing and drawing, the eChalk system is enriched by a wide range of multimedia enhancements. These may be used to enliven the lessons, allowing eChalk to surpass the didactic potentials of the traditional chalkboard. All actions on the electronic board can be tracked. The development of electronic board content can be viewed by a remote learner, both as a live transmission or as an asynchronous replay. The eChalk system allows the user to paste images from the local hard drive or from the Internet onto the board/display. These images can be loaded directly from the Web just entering their uniform resource locator (URL) during the lecture. Even better, they can be loaded using bookmarks prepared prior to the lecture. Images pasted onto the board can be annotated and edited just as if they were paper pictures stuck to a traditional blackboard. The voice of the lecturer can be recorded. In case of distance learning, the distance learner is provided with a live script where teacher's side notes are not lost. These two data streams capture most of the substance of the lecture. Optionally, a video stream of the teacher can be added to provide a more personal touch to the remote lesson.

In order to use the eChalk software in the classroom, teachers need a pen-based input device and wide display. Following alternative device configurations (display device) are in use:

1) *Digitizer tablets or tablet PCs with LCD projector*: The lecturer writes in a tablet while the computer screen is projected by a beamer. The advantages of this configuration are: *a*) digitizing tablets are comparatively affordable and easy to transport, *b*) if a tablet with integrated display is used, the lecturer can face the audience while writing, *c*) support interaction with the students through eye contact, and *d*) this medium is highly mobile.
2) *Digitizing whiteboards*: These are wide, vertically mounted digitizing tablets (up to 803 diagonal). The screen content is displayed on the surface by an LCD projector. Advantages of this configuration are: *a*) the lecture is displayed in the same spot as it is developed further focusing the attention of the audience and *b*) this configuration provide wider movements for teachers while working at the board, keeping them more active than in the tablet setup. Disadvantages of this configuration are: *a*) the lecturer often cast shadows on the projection, *b*) even slight movements of non-fixed white board or projector require the pen settings to be recalibrated and *c*) when teachers turn to the students, they might look into the projection beam.
3) *Retro projectors with pen tracking*: The key advantage of using a retro projection system is that nothing interferes with the projection beam. Because contrast and luminance are much better than those of an LCD projector. These are usable without darkening the room. Heavy weight, bulkiness and high unit costs

are the three disadvantages associated with the retro projectors.

All the three configurations (setups) are restricted by the limited size of writing area and the low resolution of the displays. While the described digitizer hardware is theoretically capable of recognizing the pen's location far beyond the accuracy of the human hand, the resolution is limited by the screen resolution of the projector and the controlling computer's graphics card. However, organic displays might solve these problems as very wide and high-resolution screens are expected to be available within the next few years.

d) *Episcope, microprojector, direct projector, and 35 mm slide projector*: These devices became obsolete after introducing the LCD projector. Compared to LCD projector, these devices are very expensive and give less presentation clarity. Mini slide projector (35 mm slide projector) is used to project 35 mm photographic slides. Slides preparation for these devices is time consuming and expensive. Episcope is used to project diagrams, pictures and other material from text books. Microprojector is used to project the microscopic slides. Direct projector has combined functions of episcope and overhead projector. This is used for projection of transparencies, printed matter and three dimensional objects.

2) **Audio aids:** Film, video, television broadcast, audio and video teleconferencing, and some computer-assisted instruction, employ audio as an integral medium. Audio medium is used to reinforce the given sound and also has a vast number of practical and innovative opportunities in distance education such as telecommunication. With audio tape/CD or radio delivery modes, audio stands alone and may be categorized as 'little media'. If the audio is combined with other modes

of visual presentation (e.g., film, video etc.) and delivered by expensive hardware, it becomes an integrated component of large medium.

A) ***Public address system***: Public address (PA) system is an electronic amplification system consisting of mixer, amplifier and loudspeakers, used to reinforce a given sound. The simple PA system consists of a microphone, modestly-powered mixer-amplifier (which incorporates a mixer and an amplifier in a single cabinet) and one or more loudspeaker. Simple PA system provides 50 to 200 watts of power and is used in small venues such as college/university auditorium. Since the PA system reinforces the sound, this medium is mainly used to make the lecture/presentation to a large group. The disadvantage of this method is that it requires uninterrupted electricity and technical assistance.

B) ***Audio tape/audio CD***: The simple audio tape and its newer version CD are also used in teaching-learning. Audiotape is a magnetic sound recording format and CD is an optical disc used for recording. Audio tapes have become outdated after the invention of audio CD. Recorded voice is also used for narration while presenting slides, films and pictures. Audio medium is widely used in distant education and self-learning. For distance education, the regular lectures are recorded or specially created.

Advantages

1) It can be designed to be used on its own or with visuals.
2) Less expensive.
3) Very portable, enables distance students to listen wherever they have access to cassette player/CD player.

3) Audio visual aids

A) Video tape/video CD: Videotaped lectures add the sense to sight in the learning experience. Videotape is a means of recording images and sound onto magnetic tape/CD. Videotape is older type and has become outdated after the invention of video CD. Video tape/ video CD medium may be used to introduce a new topic or show some pictures related to topic during the lecture/presentation. Videotapes are useful for presenting the information in didactic teaching, thereby triggering discussion. Videotapes are also useful tools for direct self-observation and feedback. This medium is useful for distant learning and videoconferencing. For distant learning, regular lectures are recorded or specially created for display.

B) Virtual reality: It is a specific computer-based technology tool (multimedia) or an interactive learning environment that is extremely close to *reality* which give the illusion of being immersed in a 3-dimensional (3D) space with the ability to interact with this 3D space. In the virtual reality world, the users believe that what they are doing is *real,* even though it is an artificially simulated phenomenon. Virtual reality learning is "best used to give students experiences of things they cannot experience in the real world, like the inside of an atom".

The interface hardware components consist of a visual display apparatus, input device and position sensor. Helmet is used as a visual display apparatus. This places a television-like screen over each eye, blocking one's view of the physical world. Instead of the physical world, student sees a 3D version of a place that is created by computer graphics. Input devices range from a keyboard to a mouse to a wand to a fiber optic glove. The purpose of the input device is to allow the human participant to give electrical signals to the computer which can be interpreted as specific commands. Depending on how the software was programmed, student mouse button or hand gesture might represent "fly forward" while another button or gesture means "fly backward."

There are two distinct categories of virtual reality systems. These are immersive (which is based on helmet-mounted or immersive display technologies) and non-immersive (which presents images on a normal monitor and allows the user to interact with the computer-generated images. Although the user is not technically immersed, it is considered as a virtual reality system because it is comparable to viewing a real world through a window) virtual reality or desktop virtual reality.

4) **Written aids:** Handouts or written aids are the form of written communication. Handouts contain the information/details on the lecture to be given or given lecture and are provided to the students for further reference. Importantly, the handouts should: *a*) contain the information/details which are not available in the textbooks, *b*) be as brief as possible, *c*) be easy to understand and *d*) be meaningful to the reader. The contents of handout should be relevant to the lecture but should not repeat the entire lecture/presentation. Two types of written handouts can be prepared. These are completed (contains all the information about the lecture with additional information and references) and uncompleted (contains the framework of the lecture and provides partial information, which has to be completed by the students during session) handouts. The key advantage of this medium (written handouts) is that it gives information about the lecture and can be used as a reading material and reference after the lecture.

5) **Patients and real objects:** Patients are used as teaching-learning medium in medical and paramedical education.

This medium provides direct interaction with patients, a better approach to learn the practical problems. For example, patients are the ideal medium for learning medical and pharmacy (clinical and community pharmacy) aspects. In particular, to teach-learn the clinical manifestations, natural history of the disease, diagnostic and therapeutic problem solving, patient counseling and communication skills with patients efficiently, patients are highly essential. This medium is suitable for only small group teaching-learning. If the study involves a rare disease/aspect, sufficient patients may not be available. In such cases, other media can be used with this medium. Real objects such as anatomical and pathological specimens and histological and histopathological section slides are the suitable media to teach-learn the anatomy and pathology aspects. Real objects are more appropriate for learning the operating procedures of equipments and instruments.

6) Three dimensional objects

A) Models: If the real objects or specimens are not available to explain the structures and functions of the human body organs and systems, models are ideal substitute in teaching-learning the anatomy and pathology aspects. Basically, model is a simplified abstract view of the complex reality in three dimensional representations. Models are suitable to teach about different organs and systems of the human body and molecular structures of chemical compounds.

B) Simulators: Simulators are functional models, used in many contexts, including the human systems and equipments in order to gain insight into their functioning. This medium is appropriate for teaching-learning psychomotor skills and affective domain. Simulation can be used to show the eventual real effects of alternative conditions and courses of action.

If it becomes dangerous, expensive, time consuming and difficult to learn in real life situation, this is a very useful and sometimes medium inevitable. In recent time, computer-created simulators are widely used for teaching-learning.

7) **Role-play:** Role-play is a type of simulation in which learners represent and experience specific characters of real life situation in contrived setting (e.g., patient-pharmacist and patient-doctor). This medium is useful for teaching communication skills and effective ways to interact with patients. Role-play is primarily designed to build self-experience in a safe and supportive environment. Role-play has been acknowledged as a powerful face-to-face teaching technique. Using computer and communication technologies, online role-play for distant learning can be performed through synchronous chat via webcam.

   Advantages

   1) The medium is exclusively student-centered. It supports and encourages an active learning.
   2) It supports and encourages critical thinking.
   3) It allows students to assume roles and employ a variety of skills and competencies to solve the problem.
   4) It supports and encourages knowledge transfer as the student's preconceived ideas are challenged by the position of the other characters.

8) **Mass communication:** This aid is mainly designed to teach the very large audience. It is a very popular and easy tool to reach the public.

REFERENCES

1. Adeyanju JL. 1988. The application of educational technology in pre-primary education. Journal of Educational Media and Technology 2:73-79.

2. Adeyanju JL. 1991. Production of cheap instructional materials for the 6-3-3-4 system of education with emphasis on the first six years. Trends and Research in Educational Technology 45-53.
3. Griggs T. 2001. Teaching as acting: Considering acting as epistemology and its use in teaching and teacher preparation. Teacher Education Quarterly 28:23-37.
4. Murphy K. 2001. Role-plays, panel discussions and simulations: Project-based learning in a web-based course. Educational Media International 38:261-70.
5. Friedland G, Knipping L, Schulte J, Tapia E. 2004. E-Chalk: A lecture recording system using the chalkboard metaphor. Interactive Technology and Smart Education 1:9-20.
6. E-Chalk. http://www.echalk.de.
7. Dickey MD. 2003. Teaching in 3D: Pedagogical affordances and constraints of 3D virtual words for synchronous distance learning. Distance Education 24:105-121.
8. Burdea GC. 2004. Teaching virtual reality: Why and how? Presence 13:463-483.
9. Smedley TM, Higgins K. 2005. Virtual technology: Brining the world into the special education classroom. Intervention in School and Clinic 41:114-119.

Chapter 17

FUNDAMENTALS OF STUDENT'S PERFORMANCE EVALUATION

Shobha Churi

"Examinations are formidable for even the best prepared, for the greatest fool may ask more than the wisest man can answer"

—J. L. Burton

STUDENT'S PERFORMANCE EVALUATION

It is a systematic process of assessment of acquisition, application and integration of subject knowledge in a competency-based curriculum. The purpose of student's performance evaluation is to determine the extent to which the general and the specific objectives of curriculum have been achieved. Student's performance evaluation is also important from the point of view of ascertaining the quality of instructional processes and to get feedback for curriculum improvement. It helps the teachers in determining the level of appropriateness of teaching experiences provided to students to meet their individual and professional needs. Evaluation also helps in diagnosing learning difficulties of the students.

Ideally, student's evaluation should incorporate periodic, psychometrically sound, comprehensive, knowledge- and performance-based formative and summative assessments, including nationally standardized assessments. To implement evaluation, two elements need to be considered. These include: intention and method of evaluation.

TYPES OF STUDENT'S PERFORMANCE EVALUATION

Evaluation is of two types: formative (internal) and summative (external) evaluation.

1) **Formative evaluation:** A progress examination can be defined as a method of assessing both the acquisition and retention of knowledge at one or more points in the curriculum relative to curricular goals and objectives. Progress examinations have been suggested for a variety of uses: *a*) peer-comparisons among institutions (also referred to as benchmarking in the educational literature), *b*) comparisons among students to identify those who could benefit from remediation, *c*) formative assessment as part of an overall assessment plan, *d*) high-stakes assessment to determine progression in the curriculum, *e*) low-stakes assessment and *f*) as an adjunct to program evaluation.

2) **Summative evaluation:** This process occurs at the end of a unit of instruction like topic, subject, semester or year. The objective of summative evaluation is to measure achievement for assigning course grades, certification of students and ascertaining accountability of instructional process. Therefore, the summative student's evaluation is required to be performed in a comprehensive and systematic manner. Any mistakes by the educators likely to affect the future of the students. Based on the summative evaluation, any educational activity can be revised, continued or terminated.

METHODS OF STUDENT'S PERFORMANCE EVALUATION

A) Based on the mode of evaluation

1) Written examinations

   a) Multiple choice questions (MCQs)-based examination

b) Essay type questions (long essay, short essay and short notes/short answers) based examination

2) Oral examinations

a) Questions

b) Higher order questions

3) Observations

a) Practical

b) Objective structured practical examination (OSPE)

c) Objective structured clinical examination (OSCE)

d) Group discussion

e) Logbook

f) Diary

B) Based on the curriculum section

1) Theory examination

2) Practical work evaluation

3) Project work evaluation

4) Professional industrial training evaluation

1) Theory examination: Theory evaluation is intended to assess student's understanding of concepts, principles and procedures related to a course/subject and their ability to apply learnt principles and solve problems. The formative evaluation of theory is carried out as sessional/class test, seminars and group discussion. The summative evaluation is conducted as written examinations. In both the cases (formative and summative evaluation), questions paper may comprise of following types of questions.

1) Multiple choice questions

2) Long essay questions

3) Short essay questions

4) Short notes/short answers

2) **Practical work evaluation:** In this evaluation, student's ability to apply or practice learnt concepts, principles and procedures, manipulative skills, ability to observe and record, ability to interpret and draw conclusions and work related attitudes are assessed. Formative and summative evaluation gives importance to performance on task, quality of product, general behavior and viva-voce.

3) **Project work evaluation:** The project work evaluation include the assessment of student's ability to apply, in an integrated manner, learnt knowledge and skills in solving real life problems, manipulative skills, ability to observe, record, creativity and communication skills. The formative and summative evaluation gives importance to nature of project, rational experimental design, product's quality, report, presentation and viva-voce.

4) **Professional industrial training evaluation:** In this process, the evaluation is performed based on student's industrial training report and viva-voce/ presentation. The objective of this evaluation process is to assess student's understanding of materials, industrial processes, practices in the industry/field and their ability to engage in activities related to problem-solving in industrial setting as well as understanding of application of learnt knowledge and skills in real life situation. The formative and summative evaluation gives importance to performance on rational approach, general behavior, quality of report and presentation during viva-voce.

MULTIPLE CHOICE QUESTIONS (MCQs) BASED EXAMINATION

A traditional multiple choice question (or item) is one in which a student chooses one or more answer or arrange answer in a required order from a number of choices provided. MCQs can be used in formative and summative evaluations. Use of MCQs concept makes the evaluation more objective type. Constructing an effective multiple choice based question paper is a crucial task, as defective MCQs are more harmful than poorly structured long essay/short essay questions, since the response is all or none in MCQs. MCQs based test is largely used to test factual material and the understanding of concepts. Because of the objectivity and ease of marking, it is frequently used for testing large groups.

Advantages

1) Can sample a broad range of course
2) Are rapidly marked
3) Students are not able to 'bluff' or 'pool' answers
4) Scoring is objective and reliable (e.g. no halo effect)
5) Distribution of scores is determined by the test not by the examiner
6) Only the objective tested are marked
7) 'Good' items may be stored in an item bank and reused

Disadvantages

1) Are time consuming to set
2) There is no credit for partial information
3) May encourage guessing
4) Good MCQs tests are difficult to set
5) Student 'selects' information
6) May encourage reproduction learning

Structure of MCQs

MCQs generally consist of following parts.

- *Stem*-question or incomplete statement
- ***Options***-suggested answers or completions

- *The key*-correct response
- *Distracters*-incorrect responses

Types of MCQs

The MCQs are classified as follows.

1) ***Single response type***: Are the traditional choose one from list of options

   Example: Which one of the following drugs is used to treat Rheumatoid Arthritis?

   a) Metformin

   b) Methyldopa

   c) Methotrexate

   d) Meropenam

2) ***Multiple response questions (MRQs)***: These are similar to MCQs, but involve selection of more than one answer from the options supplied.

   Example: Which are the following parameters used to check the renal function?

   a) Serum creatinine

   b) Blood glucose

   c) Blood urea nitrogen

   d) Serum cholesterol

3) ***Multiple true/false questions***: These questions require a student to assess whether each of the options given is true or false in association to the item. Each of the option may be true or false and are not interdependent.

   Example: A 28 year old woman with one child has taken anti-thyroid drugs for 6 months for thyrotoxicosis. She has a friend who has been successfully treated with radio-iodine. She finds she frequently forgets to take her drugs and wants to stop them to have radio-iodine treatment.

a) She should be told that because of her age radio-iodine is best avoided

b) The problems associated with radio-iodine should be discussed with her

c) Surgery as a possible alternative should be discussed with her

d) She should be advised that some form of further treatment is required

e) You should find out more about her friend's treatment

4) ***Assertion-reason questions***: This type of questions are used to explore whether each statement is correct and then to determine their cause-effect relationship.

Example: The blood sugar level falls rapidly after hepactectomy

Because

The glycogen of the liver is the principal source of blood sugar

a) Both the statements are true and causally related

b) Both the statements are true but not causally related

c) The first statement is true and second false

d) The first statement is false and the second true

e) Both statements are false

5) ***Matching questions***: This type of question involves linking items in one list to items in a second list.

Example: Match the disease and the drug to treat that particular disease.

1. Diabetes mellitus	A. Chloroquine
2. Malaria	B. Omeprazole
3. Peptic ulcer disease	C. Atenolol
4. Hypertension	D. Metformin

6) ***Ranking questions/pathway questions***: This type of question requires the student to relate items in a column to one another and can be used to test the knowledge of sequences or order of events or level of gradation.

   Example: Arrange the following processes in the order in which these are performed during the preparation of tablets.

   a) Drying
   b) Granulation
   c) Punching
   d) Mixing
   e) Evaluation

Guidelines for Writing Good MCQs

Constructing good MCQs is a very difficult task. However, good MCQs can be constructed by following the guidelines given below.

1) ***Use a question format***: Item needs to be in question format rather than incomplete statement.
2) ***Avoid negative questions***: Negative question distract students from identifying correct answer.
3) ***Emphasize higher level thinking***: Use memory plus application questions which require students to recall principles, rules or facts in real life situation.
4) ***Avoid grammatical mistakes***: Use simple, precise and unambiguous wording.
5) ***Use plausible distracters (wrong response options)***: List only plausible distracters even though the number of options changes per question.
6) ***Keep option lengths similar***: Avoid making the correct answer long or short compared to other options.

7) ***Balance the placement of the correct answer*:** Correct answers needs to be placed usually as second or third option.

8) ***Avoid clues to the correct answer*:** The correct answer of one question should not be present in the stem of the other question.

9) ***Use only one correct option*:** The options should include only correct or clearly best answer.

10) ***Avoid 'all the above' option*:** Not more than two correct answers in the options are used.

11) ***Avoid 'none of the above' option*:** Cannot be assessed whether students know the correct answer in this type.

Setting of Multiple Choice Based Question Paper

Based on the number of items in a question paper and time allotted for the candidate to attempt MCQs, a multiple choice based question paper is constructed.

***Number of items*:** Sufficient number of items/questions has to be included in multiple choice based question paper to maintain validity. There is no compulsion to the number of items. However, the score obtained by the less number of items (20-30) does not signify the depth of candidate's knowledge. Therefore, about 60-90 items/questions are most favorable for 60-90 minutes examination.

***Time allotted to attempt*:** Sufficient time should be provided to the students to attempt all items in multiple choice based examinations. Provision of more time provides opportunity to guess. On the other hand, provision of less time check the student's answering pace (speedy or slow) and not the knowledge. Hence, sufficient time should be provided based on the types of MCQs, as the different type of MCQs require different time duration.

ESSAY TYPE QUESTIONS BASED EXAMINATION

Advantages

1) Compared to MCQs based assessment, essay type questions-based tests can be easily framed by the teachers.
2) Allows students for free and effective expressions.
3) Essay questions can test complex thought processes, critical thinking and problem solving skills of students.

Limitations

1) Scoring of essays is often unreliable (results cannot be duplicated in separate trials).
2) Scores not only vary across different graders but also vary with the individual grader at different times.
3) Scorers can be influenced by extraneous factors such as handwriting, color of ink and word spacing.
4) If the scorer knows the identity of the student (a poor grading practice), his/her overall impressions of that student's work will unavoidably influence the scoring of the test.
5) Canny students sometimes play on these weaknesses by learning to disguise ignorance with a cloak of flashy verbiage.
6) Essay exams place limitations on the amount of material that can be sampled in the test, a fact that may cause a student to complain (sometimes legitimately) that "I knew a lot more about the subject than the test measured".

Types of Assay Questions

1) ***Long assay***: In this section, student's in-depth knowledge, reasoning skill and organizing skill are assessed. The questions need to be well-structured,

so that students understand what is expected from them. For example, classify the types of tablets with one example. Explain in detail the processes of tablet preparation.

2) ***Short assay/short notes/short answers***: These elicit a restricted and more specific response when compared to long assay type questions. For example, define tablets. Classify the types of tablets with one example.

Guidelines for Constructing Essay Type Questions

1) ***Validity***: Based on the range of student's skills or knowledge to be tested within a stipulated time, short or long assay questions need to be designed. To evaluate whether students have developed critical thinking skills in a course, the meaning of that phrase must be clearly defined and your course objectives and essay test items should reflect the definition you have chosen. Problem-solving skills can also be tested through essay items, but the format and method for solving problems must be specified by the teacher and clearly communicated to the student.

2) ***Reliability***: Test reliability is the degree to which a test discriminates between students of differing performance levels and the consistency with which the tests are graded. Essay tests often have relatively low reliability because grading criteria can be difficult to write and many teachers don't realize that it is not only necessary to compose a model answer, but to provide students with instructions that will elicit the desired answer. The way questions are written often invites a wide variety of responses, only a few of which may reflect the criteria that the teacher intended. When teachers maintain that they must read all the essays thoroughly before they can decide on the "best" answer, it is a sure sign that their tests lack specific grading criteria and clear instructions.

3) *Grading*: Good grading practices can also increase the reliability of essay tests. Therefore, all tests should be graded anonymously to counteract the "halo effect" of a student's prior performance.

4) *Grading in large classes*: Problems with essay tests can be magnified when more than one grader is involved. Hence, in large sections, the teacher must often share the grading responsibility with other teachers. Therefore, it is crucial that teacher follow the designed guidelines for test construction and grading.

REFERENCES

1. Newble DI, Jaeger K. 1983. The effect of assessments and examinations on the learning of medical students. Medical Education 17:165-171.
2. Rademakers J, Ten Cate TJ, Bar PR. 2005. Progress testing with short answer questions. Medical Teacher 27:578-582.
3. Kellagan T, Stufflebeam D, Wingate L (Eds.). 2003. International handbook of educational evaluation. Kluwer Academic, Dordrecht.
4. Madaus G, Scriven M, Stufflebeam D (Eds.). 2003. Evaluation Models: Viewpoints on educational and human service evaluation. Kluwer-Nijhoff, Boston, MA, USA.
5. Rossi P, Lipsey M, Freeman H. 2004. Evaluation: A systematic approach. Seventh edn. Sage Publications, Thousand Oaks, CA, USA.
6. Ware JE, Williams RG. 1975. The Dr. Fox effect: A study of lecture effectiveness and ratings of instruction. Journal of Medical Education 50:149-156.
7. Ben-David MF. 1999. Outcome-based education: Part 3- Assessment in outcome-based education. Medical Teacher 21:23-25.
8. Smith SF, Dollase RH, Boss JA. 2003. Assessing student's performances in a competency-based curriculum. Academic Medicine 78:97-107.

Section II

RESEARCH

Chapter 18
GOOD EDUCATIONAL RESEARCH PROCESS

Kashappa Goud H. Desai

"Your time is limited, but your imagination is not"

—Van Crouch

"Creative minds always have been known to survive any kind of bad training"

—Anna Freud

Research is a process of discovering or testing the hypotheses/ ideas with a method to answer a question. Identification and development of a research topic, preparation of key words/ phrases, literature review (getting an overview of the research topic), designing the rational studies/methods, obtaining the human/animal ethical approval, working, collecting and collating the data, analyzing and interpreting the data and reporting or disseminating the research data are key steps involved in the good research process.

INTRODUCTION

Research is a process of discovering or testing the hypotheses/ ideas with a method to answer a question. In other words, it is a process of establishment of facts through enquiry and exploration. The outcome of research is a new knowledge leading to improved understanding of mechanisms and the development of new and improved procedures. The purpose of research varies based on the context and so the definition of 'good' research. For example, the ultimate purpose of pharmaceutical sciences research is to create and disseminate knowledge and method to improve the human health. The 'good' research is a careful and systematic process of discovering the facts or principles for the better health of humans.

STAGES OF GOOD EDUCATIONAL RESEARCH PROCESS

Following are the steps that describe effective strategies to conduct a 'good' educational research (Figure 18.1). For the easy understanding, the steps are discussed by taking an example (development of N-acetylcysteine (NAC)/poly(DL-lactide-co-glycolide) (PLGA) injectable implants) wherever necessary.

1) **Identifying and developing a research topic:** The research process begins with deciding about a research topic. Following are tips to identify and develop an idea into a research question.

   a) Decide on a general area of interest (e.g., development of PLGA injectable implants).

   b) Decide about the objective in general (e.g., the general objective may be to develop a controlled release NAC/PLGA injectable implants) and hypothesis in specific (site-specific controlled release of NAC prevent and inhibit the recurrence of head and neck cancer) terms. At this stage, it is very important to make sure that the idea/topic is novel enough to bring the new findings to the pharmaceutical science field.

   c) Once the topic is identified, discuss with advisor or reliable experts. In case of students getting an idea, make a short PowerPoint presentation to the research group, collect the suggestions and revise the objectives appropriately.

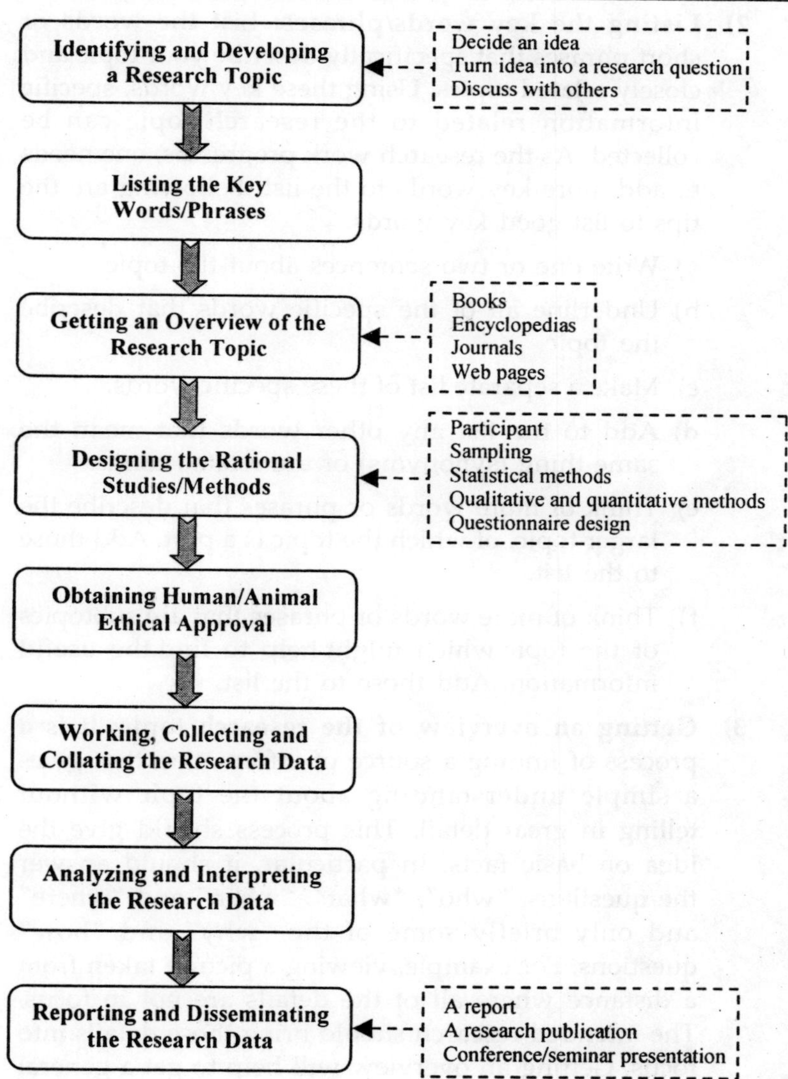

Figure 18.1. Flow of 'good' educational research process

2) **Listing the key words/phrases:** List the words or short phrases that specifically describe your topic and closely related topics. Using these key words, specific information related to the research topic can be collected. As the research work progresses, one needs to add more key words to the list. Following are the tips to list good key words.

   a) Write one or two sentences about the topic.

   b) Underline all of the specific words that describe the topic.

   c) Make a separate list of these specific words.

   d) Add to the list any other words that mean the same thing (synonyms) or are related terms.

   e) Think of more words or phrases that describe the larger topic, of which the topic is a part. Add those to the list.

   f) Think of more words or phrases that are subtopics of the topic which might help to find the useful information. Add those to the list.

3) **Getting an overview of the research topic:** It is a process of finding a source of information that gives a simple understanding about the topic without telling in great detail. This process should give the idea on basic facts. In particular, it should answer the questions: "who", "what", "when" and "where" and only briefly some of the "why" and "how" questions. For example, viewing a picture taken from a distance where all of the details are not in focus. The intended research should bring those details into focus. Getting an overview will help to get a general understanding of the topic and begin to know what kinds of subtopics are within the general topic, ask some questions that will be answered later in the research process and focus the topic into one that can be handled. Encyclopedias are one of the best

sources of overviews. Web pages, Web sites, articles and books are the other sources of information to get an overview of a research topic.

4) **Designing the rational studies/methods:** After careful consideration of the literature, rational studies/ methods that intend to answer the research question should be designed. This can be done by deciding about participant involvement (does the design methodologies pose practical or even ethical problems for those taking part), survey (if necessary, what is the most appropriate survey method for the research project), sampling (what method of sampling will give the most useful data for the project), statistical issue (familiar with the statistics you may need to use? If not, consider enrolling on a suitable course), qualitative and quantitative research methods (which are the appropriate research methods for achieving the objectives), questionnaire design (if necessary, which questionnaire is suitable) and collaboration (does the project needs or involve other research scientists/experts).

5) **Obtain human and or/animal ethical approval:** If the research methodologies involve the experiments on humans or animals, obtain the human and or/ animal ethical approval.

6) **Working on the research plan/collecting and collating the research data**

   a) One (student/trainee/researcher) should take the day-to-day responsibility and conduct the research experiments effectively. Importantly, one should ensure that research moves in the right direction (studies/methods should be relevant to the objective). Experiments that provide overflowing data/reiterate known facts should be strictly avoided. However, at this stage, if the previously designed study/method didn't fulfill the objective, alternative/modified (rational) methods can be adopted to achieve the objective. Given below is a previously mentioned example which describes how to design the rational experiments and modify appropriately based on the ongoing results.

Example: Development of controlled release NAC/ PLGA injectable implants.

To obtain one-month controlled drug release formulation, a researcher prepared 1-10 wt% NAC loaded PLGA injectable implants. Upon *in vitro* drug release studies, 10 wt% NAC/PLGA implants (a formulation with required drug content) exhibited more than 90 % drug release within 14 days, thereby suggesting the difficulty in developing one-month controlled release implant formulation for the novel anti-cancer drug (NAC). To find out the reasons for short drug-release duration, the effect of NAC on the polymer (PLGA) degradation characteristics was investigated. Interestingly, it was discovered that NAC increases the rate of PLGA degradation (determined by molecular weight decline with time), thereby exhibiting high initial burst and short drug-release duration. It is a well-known fact that an increase in the number of free carboxylic acid (COOH) groups in the polymer microclimate increases the rate of PLGA degradation. Since NAC also consist of free COOH groups, the researcher hypothesized that it might be the cause for accelerated polymer degradation and hence the short drug-release duration. To obviate this issue (high polymer degradation), the researcher formed relatively less soluble salt form of NAC (Ca^{2+} salt of NAC, where COOH group is converted to $COO^{-}Ca^{2+}$). When tested, salt form of drug (NAC-Ca^{2+})/PLGA implants exhibited slow drug release over a period of one month, thereby inhibiting the COOH induced polymer degradation. Therefore, in most cases, unexpected results open-up a new question which should be answered using the rational approaches without deviating from the principle direction.

b) Data collected in the course of research must be retained for an appropriate period of time to allow further analysis.

c) While conducting the research, take steps to seek feedback from other participants/advisor/faculty. This step allows the student/trainee/researcher to overcome the unexpected practical problems and ensure that the project runs well and meets its objectives.

d) Importantly, collected data, particularly the key breakthrough, should be kept confidentially.

7) **Analyzing and interpreting the research data:** Extensive investigation of the research problem gives large amount of qualitative and quantitative data, which should be analyzed and interpreted reasonably.

*a) **Quantitative data***: Quantitative research techniques generate a mass of numbers that should be summarized, described and analyzed. Characteristics of the data should be described and explored by drawing graphs and charts, doing cross tabulations, and calculating means and standard deviations/errors. Importantly, the figures/charts should illustrate the key findings of the research. If necessary, additional data analysis (modeling or correlations or multiple regressions or analyses of variance) should be completed.

Example: In case of a previously discussed example, the researcher conducted extensive drug stability, *in-vitro* drug release, analytical and polymer degradation experiments which provided large amount of quantitative data. Not all the data can be included in the research manuscript/ presentation. The data which adds into the manuscript's story (problem to solution) is considered as highly significant. All other relevant data should be used as supportive data.

b) ***Qualitative data:*** Qualitative data analysis describes and summarizes the mass of words generated by interviews or observational data. It allows student/trainee/researcher to seek relationship between various themes that have been identified, or relate behavior or ideas to biographical characteristics of respondents. Ultimately, theory should be developed and tested using advanced analytical techniques.

   Example: In case of a previously discussed example, the researcher used scanning electron microscopy, X-ray diffraction, fourier transform infrared spectroscopy and differential scanning colorimentry studies to understand few aspects. Instrumental results of all the formulations may not be highly necessary. Therefore, the data which proves the hypothesized theory is considered as significant.

c) ***Interpreting data***: The last step of data analysis consists of interpreting the findings to see whether they support the initial study hypotheses/findings; theory or research questions. Importantly, one should interpret the research data rationally. A story of misinterpretation: a science teacher set-up a simple experiment to show her class the 'danger of alcohol'. She set-up two glasses, one containing water, the other containing gin. Into each she dropped a worm. The worm in the water swam merrily around. The worm in the gin quickly died. "What does this experiment proves" she asked. Little Johnny from the back row piped up: "it proves that if you drink gin you won't have worms".

Following is an example of rational interpretation.

Example: In case of a previously discussed example, the researcher found following findings.

Findings

1) High initial burst effect and short drug-release duration (> 90 % drug release within 14 days) from NAC/PLGA implants.
2) Compared to blank PLGA implants, NAC/PLGA implants exhibited accelerated polymer degradation.
3) NAC-Ca^{2+}/PLGA implants exhibited slow drug release over a period of one month.
4) Slow polymer degradation of NAC-Ca^{2+}/PLGA implants over a period of one month

Interpretation: Presence of free COOH groups of NAC in the polymer microclimate increased the rate of polymer degradation and hence the drug release rate. Conversion of NAC-COOH to NAC-COO^{-} Ca^{2+} inhibited free acid induced polymer degradation, thereby providing sustained drug release over a period of one month.

8) **Reporting and disseminating the findings:** What's the next step after the data has been collected, analyzed and interpreted? The good data of the study should be used for the following purposes.

   a) ***Writing up research***: A research study report can be prepared and submitted to the concerned personnel.

b) ***Disseminating research***: The good data of research is published in the research journals.

c) ***Presentation for conferences or seminars***: The collected data can be presented in the conferences or seminars.

REFERENCES

1) Desai KGH, Mallery, SR, Schwendeman SP. 2008. Formulation and characterization of injectable poly(DL-lactide-co-glycolide) implants loaded with N-acetylcysteine, a MMP inhibitor. Pharmaceutical Research 25:586-597.

2) Giuffre M. 1996. Conducting research: Getting started. Journal of Post Anesthesia Nursing 11:104-109.

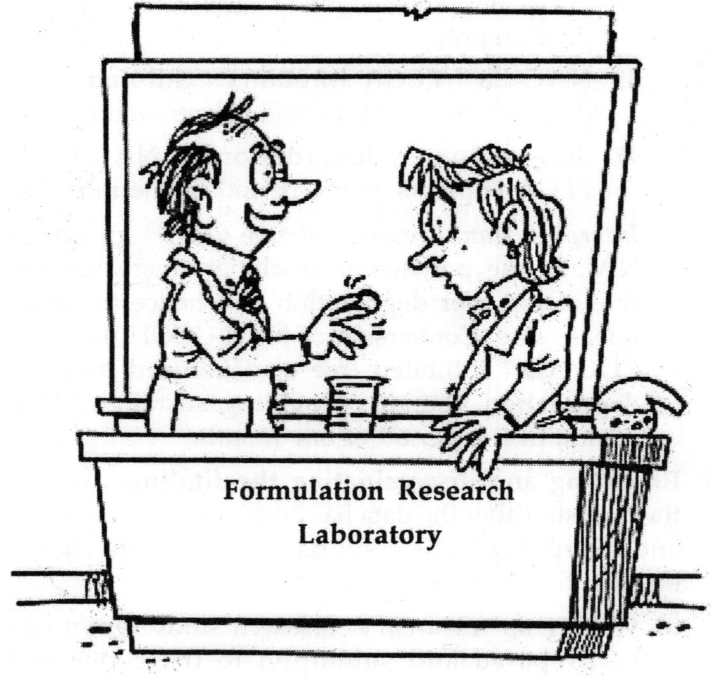

"I've done it! A cold tablet that tastes like chicken soup!"

Chapter 19

BASIC RESEARCH SKILLS, WAYS TO DEVELOP AND ASSESSMENT

Kashappa Goud H. Desai

"Creativity is a type of learning process where the teacher and student are located in the same individual"

—Arthur Koestler

A research skill is the learned capacity or talent to solve the research problem or achieve the research objective often with the minimum outlay of time, energy or both. The basic research skills are determination, curiosity, patience, enjoyment, problem formulation, finding important problems, reviewing existing work, problem solving and adaptability, self-critical eye, self-learning (lessons), independence and courage, good communication and participation in academic system. Teachers need to put significant effort to build these skills in students. Students/trainees/researchers also carry a great responsibility of involving actively in the research process and acquire these essential skills.

INTRODUCTION

Research is a process of discovering or testing the hypotheses and ideas with a method to answer a question. A research skill is the learned capacity or talent to solve the research problem or achieve the research objective often with the minimum outlay of time, energy or both. The basic research skills are required for student/trainee/researcher to conduct good educational research. These skills can be learnt or improved over a period of time. Some talent is also needed, but alone it is not enough for performing a good research. Student/trainee/researcher with great talent and no skills obtain much less success in the research than what they could do with both the qualities.

Why Do Student/Trainee/Researcher Need Basic Research Skills?

1) To learn in an analytical, synthesizing, problem solving and evaluative manner.
2) To use as scaffolding to assist learning.
3) To be prepared for the demands of the world of work.
4) To be able to learn actively, critically and reflectively.

BASIC RESEARCH SKILLS

1) Determination
2) Curiosity
3) Patience
4) Enjoyment
5) Problem formulation
6) Finding important problems
7) Reviewing existing work
8) Problem solving and adaptability
9) Self-critical eye
10) Self-learning (lessons)
11) Independence and courage
12) Good communication
13) Participation in academic system

1) **Determination:** One should have a clear and determined goal to achieve in their career/research. As a trainee, the goal should be to produce good research results and

make advancement in the field of pharmaceutical sciences. If the goal is to earn money or job promotion/increments, good research doesn't come to make advancement in the profession.

2) **Curiosity:** One should have intellectual curiosity. For example, while working on the research problem/project, one should ask some questions (how does it work? what if I change this? why did I do this?) to himself and others in all circumstances. Additionally, look what others are working/doing and learn to recognize interesting questions.

3) **Patience:** Good research needs time. Therefore, don't expect great results immediately. Experiments need to be tuned to show interesting results and lessons. Allow ample time to do theoretical or experimental research.

4) **Enjoyment:** Research career suppose to be chosen by choice not by chance. Don't do the research for money, recognition, fame and jobs. If a student/trainee/researcher likes what he does everyday in laboratory, then he should realize that this is what he suppose do in the future. Then, they are more likely to get interesting results and rest other demands/things follows the success.

5) **Problem formulation:** The research problem should be formulated in a simple and crispy manner. Everybody, even non-expert people, should be able to understand it. An unnecessary complex formulation may hide the essence of the problem and also its solution. Student/trainee/researcher can talk to others, define the problem to them and get the feedback.

6) **Finding important problems:** Working only on the current research problem/project can be useful for the next publication. But, one should devote some time also to think about the larger picture of the future research plan/problem. To do this, read relevant literature (research

work) done by other researchers and find out the important problems in the field. In case of students, they need to approach their advisor/teacher and discuss about the idea.

7) **Reviewing the existing work:** Before beginning the research project, one should be able to find and evaluate previous relevant research works. It helps to define and tune the intended research problem and obtain an idea to solve it.

   "Avoid reinventing the wheel and wasting time"

8) **Problem solving and adaptability:** Find suitable tools to answer a question or to solve a well-posed problem. One should be able to adapt to the context. For example, turn a problematic situation into an interesting research problem. If a problem arises during the course of research, then read, read and read.

   "Don't get discouraged, a solution can always be found"

9) **Self-critical eye:** If student/trainee/researcher is too sure of the research results, they will never notice the errors. If they are too unsure, they will never start the research. Therefore, errors should be considered and noted. They may be useful later to modify the theory/experiment. For example, errors can be a source of great results. Allow others to sit for your research work presentation and take the suggestions and comments positively.

   "There is always something you can learn from others"

10) **Self-learning (lessons):** In the research, a system or tool may be a useful object, and experiments may be good, but what is most important is the general lesson learnt by developing it. One should use this lesson to build different tools or define other experiments. Further, student/trainee/researcher needs to learn from failures (or from rejected papers). Work hard on your specific propagator, but think about the general consequences of your results.

"Work locally, think globally"

11) **Independence and courage:** Besides listening to or discussing with other researchers, one should also have independent thoughts. Further, they should also have courage to pursue their ideas which in turn requires self-confidence and courage to know when to stop. Don't worry to state your ideas and to be criticized. Remember that it's better to be criticized than to be ignored.

12) **Good communication:** Once the required research is completed, the research data is intended to be published as research paper or written as a thesis/dissertation or given as oral or poster presentation. Therefore, one should be able to perform all of these functions effectively.

    "Idea and motivation are important, not just the technical details"

    "The simpler is the way to present the idea, more likely to get spectators/reviewer's attention"

13) **Participation in academic system:** One should write reviews, maintain good reputation among the community and have a good attitude.

GENERAL RECOMMENDATIONS

1) **Work hard:** Student/trainee/researcher needs to work very hard to achieve the goals.

    "Given two people with equal abilities, the one who works 10 % more will produce twice as much"

    "The more you know, the more (and faster) you learn, the more you can do"

2) **Drive and commitment:** Student/trainee/researcher should be committed to the assigned research work/ project. The research is not a 9 to 5 employment. It should not be a sacrifice, but an opportunity to do something you enjoy.

3) **Openness to other students/researchers/faculty:** Student/ trainee/researcher should be open to others and to other's work. Further, they need to read and discuss a lot with others.

"Student/trainee/researcher who work with a closed door produce more in the short term but obtain less, and less interesting results, in the long term"

4) **Collaboration:** Collaborating with others lead to more than one point-of-view, faster definition of the problem and easy solving of the problem through more techniques.

   "Great work comes out of collaborations with others"

5) **Trust the advisor:** Students should trust their advisor(s). He is largely judged by the success of his students. Advisor(s) gets great inspiration by working with students. Advisor(s) learns a lot from students.

6) **Be open to many diverse experiences:** Student/trainee/researcher should take different courses, go to conferences, and spend periods in industry or other laboratories.

DEVELOPING BASIC RESEARCH SKILLS IN STUDENTS

In the current scenario, education is being directed towards new goals (skills), views of teaching and learning (constructivist) and assessment strategies (performance and authentic assessment). Skills are increasingly becoming necessary for students to perform well during the course of education as well as in the career.

Therefore, teachers carry great responsibility of building/developing the basic research skills in students. Development of basic research skills in students involves two key steps: integration of essential elements and building the development of research skills. The three essential elements of research skills which are required to be integrated in the initial learning process are depicted in Figure 19.1.

Integration of Essential Elements of Research Skills

- Teachers need to supply relevant knowledge needed to master the procedures, processes and techniques.

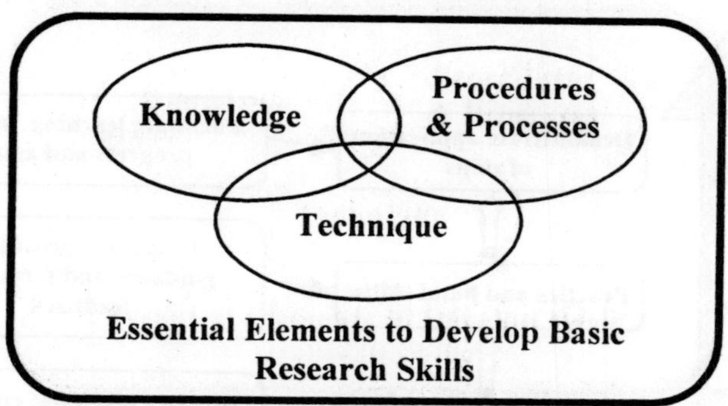

Figure 19.1. Essential elements to develop basic research skills

- Teachers need to supply the steps for and an explanation of the procedure/process/ technique(s).
- Teachers need to supply a learning task to apply and hone/refine the relevant procedure/process/ technique(s).
  a) Guided practice exercises to master the steps of the procedure/process/technique(s)
  b) Autonomous practice opportunities to refine the procedure/process/technique(s)
  c) Assessment of progress with feedback on level of mastery
  d) Opportunity to reflect on own learning
- Final summative assessment of mastery
- Other peripheral issues like motivation, learning ability, etc are naturally part of the learning process.
- Roles of teacher and student's continuum of skill development is depicted below (Figure 19.2).

Building the Development of Research Skills into Learning Opportunities

Following are the key tasks to be performed by the teachers to build the development of research skills in students.

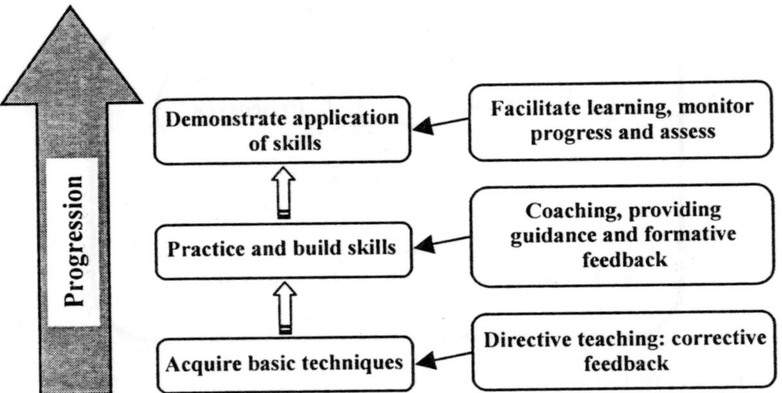

Figure 19.2. Schematic representation of student's continuum of skill development

- Supply structured guidelines on applying the skills.
- Be clear about intended student's outcome. Teachers need to know few aspects as mentioned below
  a) What do you want the student to be able to do?
  b) What does the student need to know in order to do this well?
  c) What activity will facilitate the learning?
  d) How will the student demonstrate the learning?
  e) How will I know the student has done this well?
- Determine which of the skills are relevant for a specific assignment and determine how these skills can be part of the assignment.
- Build the assignments around specific research skills. The design of the assignment should be such that it incorporates the use of a range of information formats and search strategies and encourages the evaluation of the sources that are used.
- Break down the assignment into research strategy steps. Further, break up the assignments into achievable

segments with set due dates that require the student to reflect on his process.

- Make skills a part of competence-based learning tasks in the classroom.
- Define the standards by which student's final products will be judged.
- Encourage evaluation of the process and the results at each step. Give credit for and grade each step
- Students need to create a portfolio or research log of his/her process.

ASSESSMENT OF STUDENT'S RESEARCH SKILLS

Teachers must make number of choices. The criteria of assessment are dependent on the research steps or skills that may be emphasized and the teacher's goals. Regarding scoring, teachers must make choices about how much to take into account any assistance that may have been received by the student and how to keep sight of individual performance when assessing group products and they must decide how to combine sub-scores. Teachers must also develop norms for the performance level that is to be regarded as satisfactory. Finally, teachers must register and communicate their approach and the results, and they must be accountable to students, parents, colleagues and the institution administration.

REFERENCES

1. Lock R. 1989. Assessment of practical skills. Part 1. The relationships between component skills. Research in Science and Technological Education 7:221-233.
2. Hodson D. 1992. Assessment of practical work. Science and Education 1:115-144.
3. Alexander PA, Schallert DL, Hare VC. 1991. Coming to terms: How researchers in learning and literacy talk about knowledge. Review of Educational Research 61: 315-343.

4. Anderson JR. 1982. Acquisition of cognitive skill. Psychological Review 89:369-406.

5. Haertel E. 1985. Construct validity and criterion-referenced testing. Review of Educational Research 55:23-46.

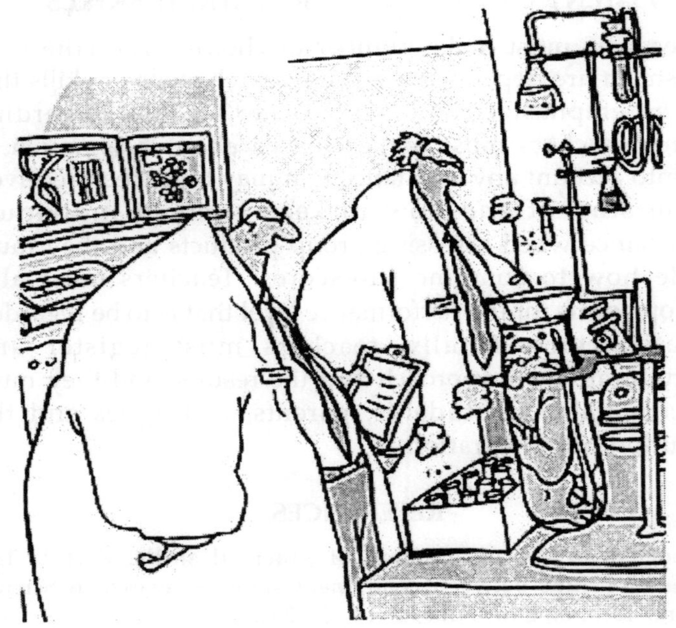

"Nobody's perfect, but we're working on it."

Chapter 20

BASICS OF GUIDING/ MENTORING STUDENTS

Kashappa Goud H. Desai

"To grow, you must get out of your comfort zone"

— Robert J. Wemecke

"Mentor should never notice what has been done. See what remains to be done"

Guiding/mentoring is a close and individualized relationship that develops over time between a student and faculty member and includes both caring and guidance. Anyone who wants to be good mentor/advisor should have the basic characteristics (great generosity, patience, perseverance, joy and enthusiasm, confidence, thoughtful planning and willingness to study). Mentor/advisor should engage students in ongoing conversations, demystify institution, provide constructive and supportive feedback, provide encouragement and support, help foster networks, look out for the student's interests, treat students with respect and provide a personal touch to exhibit effective mentorship.

INTRODUCTION

Teaching and guiding/mentoring have found a great deal of appreciation among students, whose needs have changed. The complexity of the knowledge based global economy, with its wealth of information and opportunities, has increased student's desire for help: the more decisions they have to make, the more guidance they want.

Guiding/mentoring is a close and individualized relationship that develops over time between a student and a faculty member and includes both caring and guidance. Although there is a connection between mentor and advisor, not all mentors are advisors and not all advisors are mentors.

LEVELS OF LEARNING PROCESS IN RESEARCH

There are five levels of learning at the research university: lower division, upper division, master, doctoral and postdoctoral. Research is undertaken at each of these levels, from lower division (where students learn the most basic research skills) to postdoctoral (where they acquire the most advanced research expertise). Therefore, universities/institutions need to take into consideration the complex educational requirements of today's students and provide them with training commensurate with their needs. The needs of students can only be fulfilled through effective guiding/mentoring by the faculty.

ESSENTIAL CHARACTERISTICS OF GOOD MENTOR/ ADVISOR

Mentor/advisor should:

1) be generous
2) have great patience
3) have great perseverance
4) be highly enthusiastic and enjoy mentoring
5) have great confidence
6) be able to make thoughtful planning
7) exhibit willingness to study and spend time to identify the needs of the student/researcher

ROLES OF ADVISOR/MENTOR

- Evaluate student's/trainee's skills.
- Encourage student's/trainee's growth.

- Offer opportunities to student/trainee for improvement.
- Offer professional career advice to student/trainee.
- Share their thoughts and professional values with student/trainee.
- Express and act on their commitment to mentoring.

BENEFITS OF MENTORING: STUDENT'S POINT-OF-VIEW

- Mentoring/guiding enables student/trainee to acquire the body of knowledge and skills they need.
- It also enables student/trainee to acquire an understanding of the way their discipline operates.
- Student/trainee exhibit higher productivity levels, a higher level of involvement with their departments, and greater satisfaction with their programs.

BENEFITS OF MENTORING: FACULTY POINT-OF-VIEW

- Keeps abreast of new knowledge and techniques.
- Gain collaborators for current or future projects.
- Allows to have research assistants whose work is critical to the completion of a research grant
- Gain increased professional stature by sending new scholars into the field
- Experience the personal joys and satisfactions inherent in mentoring relationships

GOOD PRACTICES OF GUIDING/MENTORING

Following are key tasks/good practices of a mentor/ advisor.

1) **Engage students in ongoing conversations**

- Mentor/advisor needs to spend time talking with student/trainee.

- Ask a student/trainee about his or her courses or current work.
- Let students know they are welcome to talk during the office hours.

2) Demystify institution

- Advisor/mentor needs to explain and guide the students about academic selections, scientific terminologies, teaching and research.
- In addition, advisor/mentor needs to explain clearly about their expectations from student.

3) Provide constructive and supportive feedback

- Advisor/mentor needs to explain and guide the students about academic selections, scientific terminologies, teaching and research.
- Advisor/mentor needs to provide students with forthright assessments of their work.
- Do not assume that students know what you think about their work.
- In addition, advisor/mentor needs to provide feedback on student's work in a timely manner, temper criticisms with praise when it is deserved and discuss with students regularly to share and solve their problems/questions.
- If students are not doing well with the research, do not doubt the student's capability instantly. Instead, address the problems and solve them.

4) Provide encouragement and support

- Advisor/mentor needs to encourage students to discuss their ideas, even though the ideas are naive or 'crazy.'
- Advisor/mentor should encourage students to try new techniques and expand their skills.

- Let students know it is okay to make mistakes. But, suggest learning from their mistakes/failures.
- Try to boost the student's confidence by assuring them that they have the skills and abilities to succeed.
- Teach students how to break large tasks into smaller ones to avoid being overwhelmed by the nature of course work.

5) Help foster networks

- If advisor/mentor is not in a situation to help/provide the student's need, then suggest other people who might be of assistance.
- Advisor/mentor should introduce the students to other faculty and students (within and outside the college and conferences) who have complementary interests.

6) Look out for the student's interests

- Let your students know up front that you want them to succeed.
- Create opportunities for students to demonstrate their competencies. For instance, take your students to important meetings and conferences so they can gain some visibility. Encourage them to make presentations at these venues.
- When you feel a student is prepared, suggest or nominate him or her for fellowships, projects and teaching opportunities.
- Be an advocate for a student if and when this is necessary.
- Promote the student's work within and outside your department.

7) Treat students with respect

- Students often feel they are not getting full attention of the mentor/advisor while talking or working on the research project. Therefore, advisor/mentor needs to give full attention while talking or discussing about research progress. Minimize interruptions during meetings. It's good idea to meet students for a coffee/tea and discuss about the research progress.

- Maintain notes on discussions with students and then file them away in a folder separate from a student's official record. Advisor/mentor needs to review these files prior to advisor-student meetings.
- Advisor/mentor is also a learner and learns from their students. Convey this fact to the students which makes them to realize they are potential colleagues.
- Acknowledge the skills and experience students bring with them to institution.

8) Provide a personal touch

- Students may face certain academic and nonacademic issues while they are in institution. Students may feel to share with advisor and try to approach for the solution/suggestion/care. Therefore, recognize the student's need and assist them in finding creative solutions to issues.

REFERENCES

1. Adams HG. 1992. Mentoring: An essential factor in the doctoral process for minority students. The GEM Program, Notre Dame.
2. Gaffney NA. (Ed.). 1995. A conversation about mentoring: Trends and models. Washington, DC: Council of graduate schools.
3. Wayne state university graduate school. 1992. Handbook for advising doctoral students.
4. http://www.rackham.umich.edu/student_life/Publications/StudentMentoring/mentoring.pdf/
5. http://www.sgs.utoronto.ca/current/supervision/guidelines.pdf

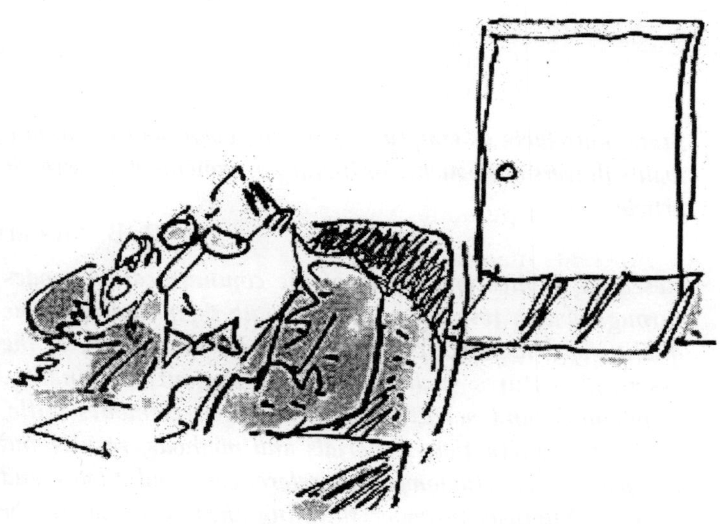

"Your thesis on "how to keep warm in winter"? Interesting."

Chapter 21
ART OF WRITING GOOD SCIENTIFIC MANUSCRIPT/PAPER

Kashappa Goud H. Desai

State your facts as simply as possible, even boldly. No one wants flowers of eloquence or literary ornaments in a research article.

—R. B. McKerrow

Research publication is one of the communication modes through which researchers disseminate their findings. The quality of a manuscript is governed by the quality of the essential features such as research content (originality, importance and scientific validity), key elements (title, abstract, introduction, materials and methods, results and discussion, conclusions, and references) and tables and figures. Manuscript/paper fulfilling these criteria can be regarded as a 'good' scientific manuscript/paper.

INTRODUCTION

The advancement of science becomes easier when the research findings are effectively and widely communicated. The researchers mainly disseminate their findings through research publications, thereby contributing to the advancement of science. Research contribution may be the prime criteria while securing and retaining the faculty position in the university/institution. The research contribution of a researcher is mainly analyzed by the quality of his/her publications. As a result, there has been significant increase in the competition among the researchers to publish high-quality research papers, thereby increasing the flow of papers to the journals. Editors, set with a task of increasing the impact factor of the journals, often reject huge number of papers due to lack of novelty in research and good writing. Therefore, researcher/faculty needs to know not only conducting high-quality research but also effective writing skills. However, writing a good scientific manuscript is a challenging task for the faculty/researcher. To publish, one has to be able to write a scientific manuscript in a format that the readers and the reviewers can follow and learn from it. One should develop spontaneous writing, creating/ adhering to self-imposed timelines and efficient writing abilities. Following are the essential guidelines that should be considered, applied and followed to prepare a good scientific manuscript/paper.

QUALITIES OF GOOD SCIENTIFIC MANUSCRIPT/ PAPER

Important qualities of a good scientific manuscript/paper are research content and presentation style of key elements and tables and figures. The qualities are discussed below. Faculty/researcher needs to prepare the manuscript/paper by incorporating these qualities. With these qualities, manuscript is more likely to get publish in the good impact factor journals.

A) **Research content:** All the material of the research (what, why and how you did it, results and their interpretation and what you concluded) is called as research content of the scientific paper. The rejection or acceptance of a paper is mainly determined by the quality of the research content. The reviewers and editor of the journal assess the quality of the research content on the basis of originality, importance and scientific validity. Therefore, before writing a manuscript, faculty/researcher needs to assess the quality of the performed research. If the student's research findings are unoriginal, unimportant or scientifically flawed, then faculty must insist to acquire high-quality research content.

1) ***Originality***: The performed research should add/ contribute to the knowledge in a material way or move the subject matter further forward. Research that confirms the findings of others may still be original. Differences in laboratory methods may also be relevant in confirming the findings of others while retaining originality.

2) ***Importance***: This is a relative and some degree subjective notion. All the original discoveries are important, because they expand the knowledge base regardless of their implications, which at first may be unclear.

3) ***Scientific validity***: In a research, rational methods and reasonable results assessment should be adopted. If a manuscript doesn't fulfill these two criteria, paper will likely to get criticism on the methods or the analysis of the results. In this context, faculty may get an opportunity to re-analyze the results, perhaps using more appropriate statistical tests. However, the methods cannot be changed without re-doing the research. Hence, if anyone has any question/ doubts, it is better to clarify/seek advice beforehand.

B) **Presentation of key elements:** Presentation style of key elements play crucial role in publishing a paper. The objective of writing a paper is to communicate precisely to readers. Precise communication can occur only when the readers understand the research content in the way it was intended. Therefore, authors need to understand/ catch the reader's expectation on information presentation.

Ideally, the scientific papers are presented in sections: title, authorship, abstract, introduction, materials and methods, results and discussion, conclusions, acknowledgements and references (see Figure 21.1). The material in each of these sections should serve a distinct purpose. Information from one section is retained as the next section is read, and so the reader also expects a logical and understandable link between the sections.

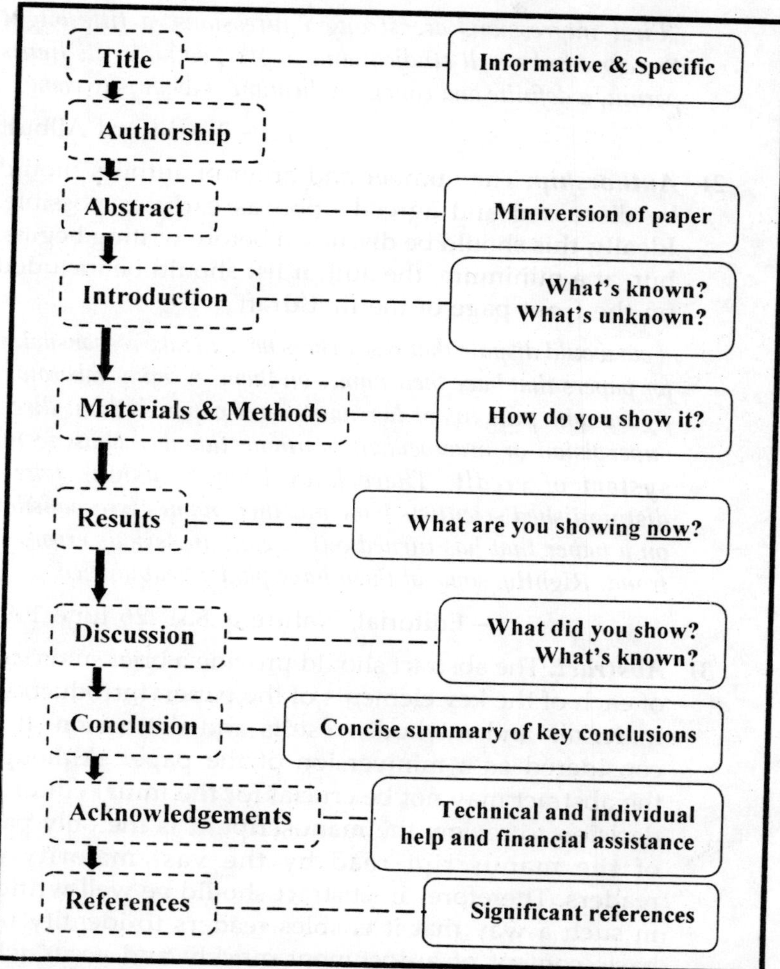

Figure 21.1. Structure of a scientific manuscript. Key elements of a scientific manuscript is depicted

1) ***Title***: Title should contain fewest possible words and adequately describe the contents of the paper. Too short or too long title is not appropriate for a scientific manuscript. Therefore, title should be informative and specific to the study and contain key elements that present the paper's contents.

"First impressions are strong impressions; a title ought therefore to be well studied, and to give, so far as its limits permit, a definite and concise indication of what is to come"

—T. Clifford Allbutt

2) ***Authorship***: The number and order of authors should be discussed and agreed upon as early as possible. Ideally, this should be discussed before writing begins, but, at a minimum, the author list should be included on the front page of the first draft.

Few would dispute that researchers have to take responsibility for papers that have their names on them. A senior laboratory figure who puts his or her name on a paper without direct supervision or involvement is unquestionably abusing the system of credit. There have been occasions where distinguished scientists have put their names irresponsibly on a paper that has turned out to contain serious errors or fraud. Rightly, some of them have paid a heavy price.

—Editorial, Nature, p.831, 26 June 1997

3) ***Abstract***: The abstract should provide a brief summary of each of the key elements of the paper: introduction, materials and methods, results and discussion. It is considered as a miniversion of the paper. Although the abstract may not be crucial for the initial editorial decision to review the manuscript, it is the only part of the manuscript read by the vast majority of readers. Therefore, an abstract should be well-written in such a way that it enables readers to identify the basic content of a document quickly and accurately, to determine its relevance to their interests.

"I have the strong impression that scientific communication is being seriously hindered by poor quality abstracts written in jargon-ridden mumbo-jumbo"

—Sheila M. McNab

4) ***Introduction***: The introduction should first contain adequate background information to allow the reader to understand and evaluate the results of the present study without needing to refer to previous publications on the topic. Then, it should state rationale for the present study. Finally, write briefly and clearly your purpose in writing the paper. Much of the introduction should be written in the present tense, because you will be referring primarily to your problem and the established knowledge relating to it at the start of your work. It is a good idea to begin writing the introduction and materials and methods sections while the work is still in progress. This makes the writing easier because everything is fresh in your mind.

"A bad beginning makes the bad ending"

—Sheila M. McNab

5) ***Materials and Methods***: In materials section, include the exact technical specifications and quantities and source or method of preparation. It is also necessary to include pertinent chemical and physical properties of the drugs, polymers, chemicals and reagents used. Avoid use of trade names. Generic or chemical name is ideal. Finally, sources of all the materials should be included.

Methods section is the active part of the paper and readers have a sense of involvement (they imagine they are doing what you have described with this section). Therefore, it is very important to present information in a logical order, usually in a chronological order. If many different procedures were used and the chronology is not crucial, then provide order for the reader by explaining each procedure under a separate sub-heading. Clarity and precision are essential. Use a flow diagram when describing a complex methodology where there are many procedural steps. The statistics used to analyze the results should be stated informatively, not simply by a list of named tests. Most of the materials and methods section should be written in past tense.

"The greatest invention of the nineteenth century was the invention of the method of invention"

—A. N. Whitehead

6) ***Results***: In this section, authors should first write the overall description of the experiments, without repeating the experimental details previously provided in materials and methods. Then, you should present the data. The results should be presented in past tense. Readers expect to see how the results accord with the aims of the study and any hypotheses that were posed. They should not have to wade through masses of disorderly information to get to this. Hence, the way of presentation of results should be planned thoughtfully. This is not easy when the research has generated numerous results. Therefore, the authors should present representative data rather than endlessly repetitive data. Authors should state the results in a simple and clear manner. Authors must avoid redundancy (repetition in words of what is already apparent to the reader from examination of the figures and tables).

"Results! Why, man, I have gotten a lot of results. I know several thousand things that won't work"

—Thomas A. Edison

7) ***Discussion***: It is the hardest section to write. Hence, many papers are rejected by journal editors because of a faulty discussion, even though the data of the

paper might be both valid and interesting. Importantly, true meaning of the data should not be obscured by the interpretation presented in the discussion. This section should contain essential features of the good discussion. Incorporation of essential features of good discussion can be achieved if the following guidelines are followed.

- Present the principles, relationships and generalizations shown by the results. In a good discussion, authors need to *discuss* not *recapitulate* the results.
- Point out any exceptions or any lack of correlation and define unsettled points.
- Show how your results and interpretations agree (or contrast) with previously published work.
- Discuss the theoretical implications of your work and any possible practical applications.
- Summarize your evidence for each conclusion.

"It is the fault of our rhetoric that we cannot strongly state one fact without seeming to be belie some other"

—Ralph Waldo Emerson

8) ***Conclusions***: The main body of the manuscript should be finished with a conclusion statement. The conclusion may be included as an integrated part of the formal discussion section or listed as a separate heading. This section should contain a concise summary of the key conclusions drawn from the current work in light of the reported findings. The author(s) need to present to the reader the relevance of the work undertaken and concisely define how this new information contributes to the existing body of knowledge. Further, recommendations for interpretation or application of the findings can also be reinforced briefly in this section.

9) ***Acknowledgements*:** Authors should acknowledge: *a*) any significant technical help received from any individual, whether in laboratory or elsewhere, *b*) the source of special equipment, cultures or other materials and *c*) any outside financial assistance, such as grants, contracts or fellowships.

"Life is not so short but that there is always time enough for courtesy"

—Ralph Waldo Emerson

10) ***References*:** References are one of the first sections read by editors and reviewers. They should be cited to support methods and claims. Authors should list the significant and published references. Avoid listing unpublished data, thesis and other secondary materials. Check all parts of every reference against the original publication before the manuscript is submitted. Finally, make sure that all the references cited in the text are indeed listed in the reference section and that all the references listed under references section are indeed cited somewhere in the text. To avoid any errors, the use of specialized reference software (e.g., Refman and End Note (Thompson Corp, Carlsbad, Calif)) is recommended.

Manuscripts containing innumerable references are more likely a sign of insecurity than a mark of scholarship"

—William C. Roberts

C) **Presentation of tables and figures:** Tables and figures should be designed according to the journal's requirement. The selection of tables and figures is done on the basis of the importance of these two representations in the current manuscript. For instance, only figures or tables which are directly related to the current study and add some benefit to the work should be included. Figures and tables that do not add direct benefit to the interpretation or understanding of the specific study being reported, even if they are of substantive or significant scientific merit, should be omitted. All figures and tables presented must be referred to at some point in the text. Any figures or tables included in the article for consideration for publication should be submitted at the end of the manuscript. Each figure or table should be provided on a separate page with its own caption (title). The caption should provide a brief description of the figure or table and clear explanation of any labels. Where the manuscript includes more than one figure or table, a summary 'captions list' should also be provided, listing the figures and tables in the order they would appear in the text.

"A tabular presentation of data is often the heart or, better, the brain, of a scientific paper"

—Peter Morgan

A good illustration can help the scientist to be heard when speaking, to be read when writing. It can help in the sharing of information with other scientists. It can help to convince granting agencies to fund the research. It can help in the teaching of students. It can help to inform the public of the value of the work.

—Mary Helen Briscoe

REFERENCES

1. Gopen GD, Swan JA. 1990. The science of scientific writing. American Scientist 78:550-558.
2. Zeiger M. 2000. Essentials of writing biomedical research papers. 2nd ed. McGraw-Hill, New York, USA.
3. Administration DoFa. 2002. Style manual for authors, editors and printers. 6th ed. Wiley and Sons, Melbourne, Australia.
4. Murray R, Moore S. 2006. The handbook of academic writing: A fresh approach. Open University Press, Maidenhead, England.

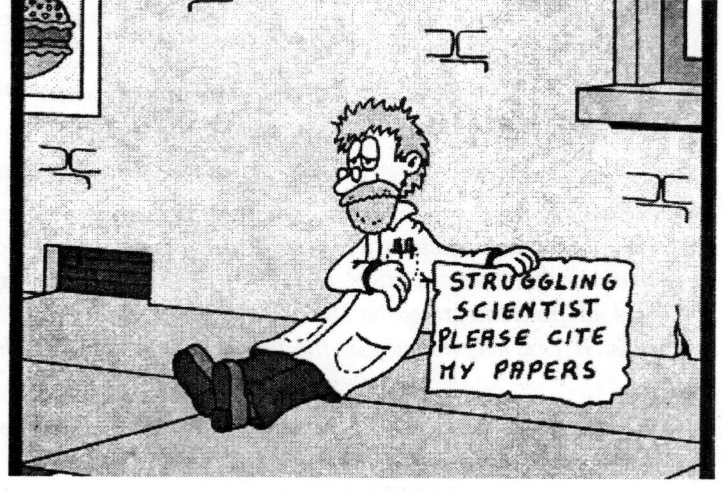
STRUGGLING
SCIENTIST
PLEASE CITE
MY PAPERS

Chapter 22
ART OF WRITING A GOOD THESIS/ DISSERTATION

Kashappa Goud H. Desai

The average thesis/dissertation (M. Pharm or Ph.D) is nothing but transference of bones from one graveyard to another.

—J. Frank Dobie

Thesis/dissertation writing is a piece of writing on the conducted research, arranged in clearly separate section(s)/ chapter(s), in which an argument (a clear line of thought) is developed in response to a central question or proposition (thesis). Thesis can be regarded as 'good' when advanced research is conducted and demonstrated (written-up) in a systematic and understandable manner. Each section/chapter of the thesis should be presented with adequate details, results and rational interpretations. This is possible only when the good research process and thesis writing practices are followed.

INTRODUCTION

Thesis/dissertation has become an increasingly important component of pharmacy education (particularly in M. Pharm and Ph. D courses) over the past few years. Students work on the research project, embed their progress/achievements in a thesis/dissertation and submit to the University. It is not just a course completion criterion. Students obtain an opportunity to work independently on an interested research project over a period of time. It is also an effective means of research training, which helps to develop advanced intellectual skills such as evaluation, analysis and synthesis, as well as management skills. During M. Pharm and Ph. D courses thesis/dissertation work, students also learn basic research skills (creative and critical thinking and problem solving skills).

Thesis/dissertation writing is a piece of writing on the conducted research, arranged in clearly separate section(s)/chapter(s), in which an argument (a clear line of thought) is developed in response to a central question or proposition (thesis). The line of argument is supported by evidence one has acquired through research. In course of argument, the gathered evidences are analyzed and evidences that support or contradict the various prospective are explored. The thesis then reaches a conclusion in the final section/final section of every chapter, which pulls together the threads of the argument, supporting, qualifying or rejecting the original thesis. Writing a good thesis/dissertation is a hard and painful work. By the time students initiate the writing of their thesis/dissertation, they must have come to the end of their research project. Some students never manage (99 % perspiration and 1 % inspiration) to write a good thesis/dissertation. Therefore, it is very crucial for the students to know about writing a good thesis/dissertation. This chapter guides through the skills of writing a good thesis so that students can easily complete this crucial responsibility.

BASIC REQUIREMENTS OF A THESIS/DISSERTATION

1) A good thesis demonstrates the student's ability to undertake a good quality research. M. Pharm thesis exemplifies the results of individual research and a Ph. D thesis represents the results of individual and novel research which makes an original contribution to scholarship. Both the theses should show evidence of a systematic study and an ability to relate the

results of the research to the general body of knowledge in that subject.

2) To ensure a measure of uniformity, there will be more specific formal requirements, which govern the length, format and presentation of theses. Find out these requirements at an early stage so that you can plan with them in mind.

3) It is recommended to get an impression of what is required by reading recent theses in the same or a comparable research area. It is much easier to emulate than it is to construct from a set of rules. However, you should be aware of two pitfalls explained below.

   a) Do not aim to produce a thesis identical in every respect to those produced previously. The thesis should be highly individual; it should contain your ideas about your original work expressed in your own way. After all, it is your own work and a document by which you will be judged.

   b) Do not assume that the likelihood of success is directly related to the length of the thesis. A thesis is read and not weighed. The thesis should be long enough to clearly and unambiguously report the results of research and discuss their significance. Since waffling and padding are easily detected by the examiners (these does not impress them), these two aspects must be avoided.

GOOD THESIS/DISSERTATION WRITING PRACTICE

Following are the effective steps and corresponding strategies to be followed for writing a 'good' thesis. The recommended format for theses is similar for most institutions with some local minor variations.

A) **Reviewing the research results:** Once the exhaustive research data is collected, students need to review the results, perform rational interpretation and reach to appropriate theory/theories on the research problem (brief summary of the conducted research). At this point, students should ensure that necessary data/graphs/tables are available to prove their hypothesis.

B) **Preparing an outline of the research work:** Students then need to prepare an outline of the whole research (step-by-step approach and obtained findings (problem to solution)). The outline should display the direction in which thesis should be written (in terms of theory, methods, discussion, conclusion and format of presentation (table of contents)). In case of Ph. D. work, more research studies are involved. Hence, a linking hypothesis between chapters/studies should be prepared. A good outline guides students through writing process efficiently.

C) **Presentation of thesis contents**

1) Title page
2) Abstract
3) Acknowledgements
4) Table of contents
5) Introduction
6) Review of the literature-concluding with a summary
7) Statement of the problem, aims of the study and hypothesis
8) Materials and methods (including statistical analysis)
9) Statistical analysis
10) Results
11) Discussion
12) Conclusions
13) Appendices
14) References

C) **Presentation of thesis contents:** The manner of writing thesis contents is described below. Also, thesis contents should appear in the order as mentioned below.

1) ***Title page***: The title page should include: *a*) title of the thesis (usually centred on the page and in upper case letters), *b*) full name and qualifications of the student, *c*) the name of the institution to which the thesis is being submitted, *d*) the degree for which the thesis is submitted and *e*) the year of submission.

2) ***Abstract***: The abstract is placed immediately following the title page and is generally short (up to a side of A4 usually). The abstract should include a: *a*) brief introduction, *b*) statement of the problem and *c*) summary of the methodology, findings and conclusions. A structured abstract may be used if preferred.

3) ***Acknowledgements***: Students need to acknowledge advisor(s), statistical adviser(s), others who have helped (e.g. colleagues who have offered support or provided data) and any funding bodies.

4) ***Table of contents***: After acknowledgements section, there should be a table of contents, followed by a list of tables and figures. The table of contents should include all the major divisions of the thesis, including subsections. The relationship between major divisions and minor subdivisions should be shown by an appropriate use of capitals and indentations. The preliminary pages (abstract, acknowledgements and contents) are numbered using roman numerals (i, ii, iii...) and the remainder of the thesis is numbered using Arabic numerals (1, 2, 3...). The title page is not numbered. The list of tables or figures follow the same format, with each table/figure number in Arabic numerals, the exact title as it appears in the main text and also the page number.

5) ***Introduction:*** In this section, one should *introduce* the thesis. Do not summarize the thesis. Importantly, it is not a brief version of each chapter. Instead, one should write an introduction to the topic (introduce the subject). In general terms, what does the study address? Why is it important? Where does is fit in the overall field? Include a clear statement of your hypothesis and how you are going to address it. The introduction should contain the citations from the research literature to support the study. These citations should include but not be limited to research presented in the literature review. The topics that are usually covered in the introduction are: *a*) statement of the problem (brief statement of the problem that your thesis is going to address with relevant information about why this is an important problem), *b*) background and need (relevant literature (research articles, books, educational and government statistics) that supports the need for your project with or without brief overviews of articles covered in the literature review that support the need for your project), *c*) rationale (the rationale should define the larger problem being investigated, summarize what is known about the problem, define the gap(s) in the knowledge, and state what needs to be done to address the gap(s)) and *d*) purpose of the project (based on the above background information, explain the purpose of the study/what you hope the study will accomplish and why you chose to do this particular study supported by the citations and specific information related to the study).

6) ***Review of the literature*:** Writing the literature review is a daunting task, particularly if you undertake extensive research. It is more appropriate to write the 'review of literature' section as soon as students complete their literature search and collect sufficient

information on the designed research project. The 'review of the literature' section should focus only on the material that gives an appropriate background to the study and be as comprehensive as possible. Students should avoid including everything they have ever read on the subject. Importantly, students need to perform regular literature search and constantly update this section till the submission of the thesis. This process updates the students on related findings and tunes their research in a better manner. Literature review section should be written with only relevant references. Great care should be taken while quoting the references in the text. If several papers are quoted at the same point, they should always be in chronological order.

7) ***Statement of the problem, aims of the study and hypothesis***: The literature review is followed by a statement of the problem, aims of the study and hypothesis. It is more appropriate to pose a hypothesis in its positive form. Students must ensure that intended hypothesis is actually answered in the results and discussion section.

8) ***Materials and methods:*** Full details of the materials, chemicals and reagents used and methods adopted should be provided in this section. The details of materials and methods should be comprehensive enough for readers to repeat the experiments identically. It is more appropriate to write this section while working on the designed experiments. This is important since everything (procedures) will be fresh in your mind at this stage and keeps the record of any modifications done during the process of study. The most serious error in this section is to omit important information required by the reader to see the logic of the study and to judge the adequacy of the method.

The details associated with the validity of the method should be given in this section. These include:

a) *Subjects:* This should include the number of subjects at each stage, freedom from bias in the way the subjects are obtained and other details of subjects (number, age group, gender, where they were recruited from, inclusion and exclusion criteria, how many subjects were asked to take part and how many agreed, drop-out rate, etc.).

b) *Design*: Design details should include what type of study was undertaken

c) *Materials, apparatus and procedures*: This part should contain the procedural elements in a manner that the readers understand these three aspects clearly. Complex procedures or mechanism of methods or apparatus should be described through the diagrams or photographs or charts.

d) *Validity and reliability*: The reliability and validity of any method should be addressed in this part. Limitations of the method should be discussed fully in the discussion section. It is better to be honest and acknowledge any issues, rather than allowing the examiner to point them out to you.

9) ***Statistical analysis***: The key research data should be treated with the suitable statistical analysis methods to find out if there is any significant difference among the methods or variables or formulations studied. The statistical tests should be discussed fully, along with any criteria that were fulfilled in order to use these tests (e.g. normality of data).

10) ***Results:*** Refer 'art of writing good scientific manuscript/paper' chapter to know about writing the results section. Research manuscript's results section contains only key results of the research. Whereas, thesis should contain relatively more results of the

research (almost every result). The results should be presented in a clear and concise manner (avoid presenting the data in more than one format (e.g., in both tables and graphs)). It is often helpful to precede each sub-section of results with a summary paragraph, but avoid duplication. Tables and figures should be as simple as possible (avoid using very complicated graphics or obscure colour combinations). Importantly, table's or figure's title should display the conditions (e.g., title of drug release plot should contain temperature value, type of release medium, pH, and formulation variables details) associated with the demonstrating study.

11) ***Discussion***: Students often find it as a most difficult task. It really is the 'thinking part' of the thesis. Refer 'art of writing good scientific manuscript/paper' chapter to know about writing the discussion section. Discussion section of the thesis should contain relatively more explanation on result's interpretation, theory and principles. It is also customary to follow the discussion with a small section on 'suggestions for further study'. This allows students to make suggestions on continuation of the study or amendments to the existing methodology.

12) ***Conclusions***: The salient conclusions from the work should be summarized in this section. Conclusions bring more impact if they are presented in bullet format. Avoid repetition and making this section too long. It is supposed to represent the most important findings, not every single finding.

13) ***Appendices***: Appendices section is used to include the data that is not required in the main body of the text or supportive details (questionnaires, patient's consent forms, information sheets given to patients, etc.) of the study.

14) *References*: Use of computer-based reference manager minimizes the errors. If you do not have access to a computer-based system for any reason, keep index cards of all the references you have read so that you can go back and double check them. This avoids a great deal of work at a later stage. Always get someone else to double check your references and cross-check that all those in the text are in the references and *vice versa*. Be consistent with the style of the references.

OTHER RECOMMENDATIONS

1) **Word limits:** Check about the word limit of thesis (M. Pharm or Ph. D) *before* initiating the writing process.
2) **Ph. D thesis:** Since the Ph. D work involves more research studies, thesis is written chapter-by-chapter (based on study-by-study). It is ideal to take a broad research problem so that a linking hypothesis can be given between chapters. Each chapter may have introduction, brief review of the literature, materials and methods, results and discussion and conclusions. Start the thesis with an overall introduction and end with overall conclusions that bring the whole thesis together.

Following are the ideal characteristics of a Ph. D work/ thesis

Ideal characteristics of Ph. D work/thesis

- Opens a new research area
- Provides unifying framework
- Resolves long-standing question
- Thoroughly explores research area
- Contradicts existing knowledge
- Experimentally validates theory
- Produces ambitious system

- Provides empirical data
- Derives superior algorithms
- Develops new methodology
- Develops new tool
- Produces negative result

3) Dealing with advisor(s): Suggestions for students

- Students should keep the relationship with advisor(s) as easy as possible during your research and throughout the writing-up phase.
- Let your advisor know how much contact and support you would like to get.
- Accept that there are limits to the amount of help that can be expected from advisor(s). Students should expect only intellectual (quality assurance, what standard a thesis should reach and indication of when to stop) and emotional (constructive atmosphere and encouragement) support from advisor(s).
- Plan together some interim deadlines for the work, so that you are able to manage your time effectively.
- Find an appropriate way of mapping and monitoring your own progress (e.g., by using a checklist of tasks to be completed). Use this to help the discussions with your advisor(s) to focus on areas where you need particular advice.
- Listen to, evaluate and respond to feedback given by the advisor(s). This can be done by making notes and reflecting on what has been said or written, then applying the feedback to the next stage of your research or writing-up.

REFERENCES

1. Van Wagenen K. 1991. Writing a thesis: Substance and style. Englewood Cliffs, Prentice Hall.

2. Anderson J, Poole M. 1998. Assignment and thesis writing. (3rd edn). John Wiley & Sons, Brisbane.

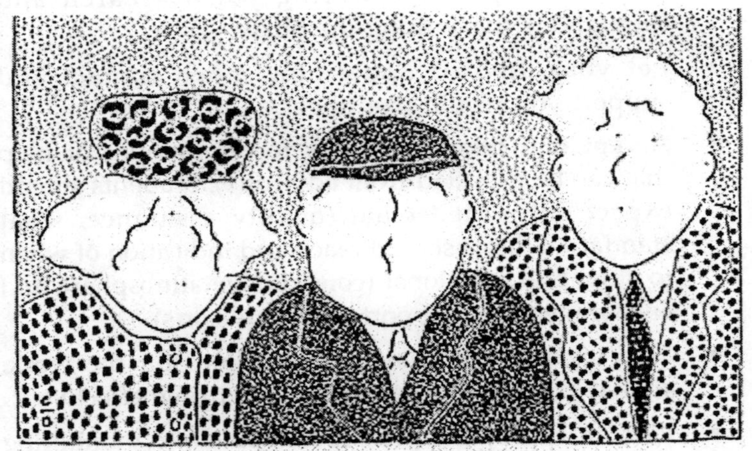

"I" am pretty sure I have a Ph. D. I think one came bundled with my new computer."

Chapter 23
HOW TO TRANSFORM A THESIS TO MANUSCRIPT(S)

Kashappa Goud H. Desai

"Many editors see themselves as gifted sculptors, attempting to turn a block of marble into a lovely statue, writers as crude chisels. In actual fact, the writers are the statues, and the editors are pigeons"

— Doug Robarchek

Theses written by the students display the research contents on the basis of university guidelines. Although the project is highly superior and bring new knowledge to the science, the editors (and reviewers) reject the thesis-style manuscripts. Step-by-step effective transformation of thesis contents can yield a good scientific manuscript/paper. While doing so, be ruthless with yourself. Otherwise, the editor and referees will certainly be much more ruthless than you.

INTRODUCTION

Thesis and research manuscript are the common modes for disseminating the research findings. Although both the forms serve the same purpose, the style of presentation of research contents between these two forms of communication is distinctly different. In thesis, students are generally allowed to describe the research contents as comprehensive as possible. In contrast, a manuscript/paper is a concise and clear dissemination report of key research findings (findings that bring new knowledge to the science). Writing a manuscript/

paper from a thesis does not mean publishing a shortened version of the thesis. Instead, students need to carefully identify and take out key research findings from the thesis. In doing so, students may have to ignore a lot of stuff of the thesis to obtain a good research manuscript. Therefore, be ruthless with yourself at the preparation level. Otherwise, the editor and referees will certainly be much more ruthless than you.

COMMON CHARACTERISTICS OF A THESIS-STYLE MANUSCRIPT

The style of thesis is suitable only for the purpose of graduation. Although the research project and its findings are strong enough for the publication in a good impact factor journal, the reviewers and editor of the journal reject the manuscript due to thesis-style presentation of the research contents. Manuscripts/papers written in a thesis style (miniversion of thesis) do not even reach the review process. Instead, editors reject them right away during the preliminary screening process. By understanding what editors (and reviewers) are seeking, authors can avoid this common problem, develop manuscript in a journal-style, save revision and enjoy the proud moment upon acceptance.

The following factors are regularly considered as clues to alert the editors that the manuscript is most likely a thesis report:

- Long title of the manuscript (like "definition")
- Long introduction and failure to justify the necessity of the paper (significance of the study or paper)
- Very long methods section. Include more number of methods (e.g., methods on measurement of thickness, hardness, disintegration of tablets etc. are not important) and methods section fail to bring focus on the key method(s) of the research.
- Very long result and discussion. Looks like a method-by-method research data report. Fail to display a good

story (from hypothesized problem to solution) of the research.

- Too much importance to statistical measures
- Very long text of the manuscript
- Practical applications of the research are short (not enough importance) or omitted.
- Not addressed to the specific needs of the readers.
- Excess and insignificant references and inappropriate style

HOW TO TRANSFORM A THESIS TO MANUSCRIPT(S)

Following are the recommendations which assist the prospective author(s) to develop a research journal-style publication from the thesis.

- Identify the key research finding(s)
- Analyze the readers of the interested journal
- Based on the key finding, develop a new outline of the research story (from problem to solution) with the appropriate headings. Avoid the typical thesis report like headings.
- Shorten the sections such as literature review, research data and theoretical framework
- Emphasize the significance of the current study or paper in the introduction with a brief summary of previous research works on the related area. Emphasize on the practical applications of the research.
- Include the (key) methods which add to the discussion and justify the major findings of the research. Do not include methods of supportive/ preliminary studies.
- Present selected results which bring sense to designed research hypothesis (story).
- Charts/graphs should display key research findings and highlight the story/hypothesis of the research.

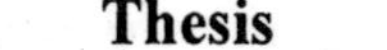

Thesis		Manuscript
• Academic writing style • Thesis heading like "definitions" • Long literature review • Focus on the past • Detailed description of statistical measures • Include almost all research data • Detailed explanation of interpretation, theories, and principles • Short implications section • Excessive number of charts and tables • Focus on institution's requirements • Excessive references • References in university's requirements • Very lengthy (60 or more pages)	Change to →	• Scholarly but not pedantic style • Heading-Short, specific and informative • Summary of past literature • Focus on the future • Explanation of statistical measures • Include key research data • Brief statements on interpretation, theories, and principles • Detailed implications section • Selected charts/tables summarize data • Target to the readers • Selected references • References in journal's style • Short (10-30 pages)

Figure 23.1. Comparison of style of presentation of research contents between thesis and manuscript.

- Provide concise and clear discussion on the results. Brief summary of relevant interpretations, theories and principles.
- If necessary, provide brief summary of the statistical measures. This can be merged with the discussion section particularly while discussing about the significant difference between the formulations or study variables or methods.
- Discuss in brief about the practical applications of the research.
- Edit the text/sections in such a way that it provides a smooth transition between titles and subtitles.
- Include only significant references and strictly follow the journal style.

The style of presentation of research contents in thesis and manuscript is compared in Figure 23.1.

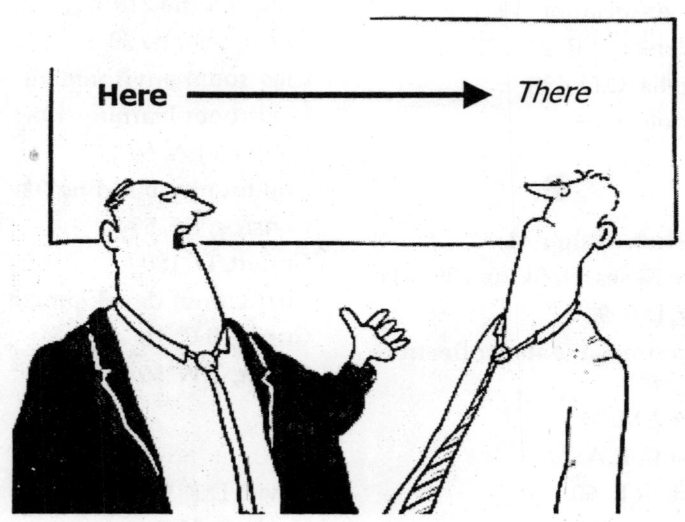

"It's a simple model......but it works for me...."

INDEX

A

Academic environment 14
Academic institutions 4
Administrators 5, 6
Aiche, J.M. 138
Alexander, P.A. 245
Allbutt, T. Clifford 258
American Pharmaceutical Association 19
Anderson, J.R. 246, 276
Angelia, C.D. 138
Atenolol 219

B

Bagehot, Walter 61
Basic Research Skills 238, 242
Beck, D.E. 94
Behavioural data collection 16
Beitz, J.M. 35
Bernoff, R.A. 11
Blake, R.L. 60
Boss, J.A. 224
Breen, R. 123
Briscoe Mary Helen 263
Brueggemeier, R.W. 59
Bucher, R. 19
Burton, J.L. 213

C

Carnes, C.A. 152
Chism, NVN 11
Chloroquine 219
Churi, Shobha 39, 61, 181, 213
Classroom environment 6
Classroom learning 128
Colliver, J.A. 60
Community building 93
Consroe, P.F. 59
Corlett, D. 180
Curriculum development 5
Currie, B.C. 76
Cutler, T.W. 59

D

David, D.K. 76
Davis, S. 180
Dawabi, P. 180

Desai, Kashappa Goud H. 12, 20, 22, 77, 81, 96, 112, 124, 139, 154, 168, 227, 237, 247, 265, 277
Devitt, P. 137
Diabetes mellitus, 219
Dobie, J. Frank 265
Dollase, R.H. 224
Downes, T. 94, 110
Drug development 131

E

Edison, Thomas A. 260
Educational evaluation 146
Educational institutions 116
Educational methodology 39
Educational productivity 82
Educational program 15
Educational Research 228
Educational technologies 96
Electronic feedback 73
Emerson, Ralph Waldo 262
Empowering teachers 87
Essential characteristics 248
Extracurricular activities 15

F

Fisher, R.C. 59
Flynn, A. 76
Freeman, H. 224
Freud, Anna 227

G

Galbraith, J.K. 81
Gather information 43, 45
Geroski, P.A. 94
Gomeni, R. 138
Goodyear, G.E. 11
Gopen, G.D. 263
Goram, A. 152
Grasha, A.F. 11
Gregory, J. 180

H

Haertel, E. 246
Hannafin, R.D. 94
Hare, V.C. 245
Haworth, I.S. 59
Herrier, R.N. 59
Hodson, D. 245
Houser, C. 180
Hussein, Y. 110
Hypertension 219

I

Individual teaching 3
Information technologies 88, 152
Internet technology 73

J

Jackson, T.R. 59
Jaeger, K. 224
James, William 181